CONTENTS.

Scientific Cooking of Vegetables
Labour-Saving Appliances
Medicinal and Dietetic Qualities of Foods
Hygienic Information
How to accumulate Physical Vitality

PREFACE TO SEVENTH EDITION.

Dietetic Reform is now being considered seriously by thoughtful people in all parts of the world and interest in this important though long neglected subject is increasing every day.

The fact that our physical, mental, and spiritual conditions are greatly influenced by the nature and quality of our daily food, and that, consequently, our welfare depends upon a wise selection of the same, is becoming generally recognized.

Popular illusions concerning the value of flesh-food have been much dispelled during recent years by revelations concerning the physical deterioration of the flesh-consuming nations, and the comparative immunity from disease of people who live on purer and more natural food; also by a succession of remarkable victories won by fruitarians who have secured numerous athletic Championships and long distance Records.

Demonstration has been provided by the Japanese, that a non-carnivorous and hygienic Race can out-march and out-fight the numerically superior forces of a colossal Empire; and that its national and social life can be characterized by conspicuous efficiency, sobriety, health, and vitality.

A vast amount of emphatic personal and medical testimony to the advantages of the more simple and natural *fruitarian* system of living is being given by thousands of witnesses who speak from experience; and such evidence is preparing the way for a complete change of popular thought and custom concerning dietetics.

In addition to such influences, an ever-increasing consciousness that the emancipation of the animal world from systematic massacre and ruthless cruelty awaits the abandonment of the carnivorous habit by the Western races of mankind, is exercising a powerful effect upon the lives of multitudes of men and women. In consequence of having reached a comparatively advanced stage of evolution, they realise the solidarity of sentient life and feel humanely disposed towards all fellow-creatures; and they cannot avoid the conviction that Man was never intended to play the part of a remorseless and bloodthirsty oppressor of the sub-human races.

Those who are labouring to bring about the adoption of dietetic customs that neither violate the physical laws of our being, nor outrage the humane sentiments of the higher part of our nature, are consequently now met by serious requests for information concerning some way of escape from bondage to ancestral barbaric custom, and the safest path to a more rational and harmonious existence. "How may we live out our full length of days in health and vigour, instead of dying of disease?" "How may we avoid the painful maladies that are prevalent, and escape the surgeon's knife?" "How may we be delivered from further participation in all this needless shedding of innocent blood?" "How may we in a scientific way feed ourselves with simple and hygienic food—with the kindly fruits of the earth instead of the flesh of murdered creatures who love life just as we do?" Such questions as these are being asked by thousands of earnest souls, and it is to help such enquirers that this Guide-Book is published.

My aim has been to give practical, reliable and up-to-date information in a concise form, avoiding superfluous matter and 'faddism,' and only supplying simple recipes which do not require the skill of a 'chef' for their interpretation. By spending a few hours in thoughtful study of the following pages, and by practising this reformed system of diet and cookery in domestic life for a few weeks, any intelligent person can master the chief principles of fruitarian dietetics, and become qualified to prepare appetising dishes suited to the taste of a hermit or a *bon vivant* (provided that its possessor be not hopelessly enamoured of the "flesh-pots of Egypt" and the flavour of cooked blood).

A system of living that is earnestly recommended by thousands of disinterested advocates who have personally tried it, that comes to us full of promise both for ourselves and others, that bids fair to humanize and transform mankind and to solve many of the world's social problems, and that is now endorsed by so many progressive medical authorities, merits such attention, and is worthy of trial.

As I am writing a *Guide* to reformed diet for domestic use—not an elaborate treatise to justify it—I have refrained from introducing medical and experimental testimony concerning the dangerous and injurious nature of flesh-food, and the advantages of living upon the fruits of the earth, supplemented by dairy products. Numerous standard works are now obtainable which demonstrate that the principles and arguments upon which the Food-Reform Movement is based are supported by an array of scientific evidence which is more than sufficient to convince any unprejudiced, logical and well-balanced mind. For such information I must refer my readers to other publications, and I have printed a short list of useful works on the final pages of this book, for the benefit of those who are as yet unacquainted with such literature.

For some of the recipes contained in the following pages I am indebted to certain of the Members of The Order of the Golden Age, and to other workers in the Food-Reform Cause—but especially to Mrs. Walter Carey, who has devoted much time to the task of preparing and testing them. Most of them are original, being the result of thoughtful experiment; and they should, *if carefully followed*, result in the production of dishes which will give satisfaction. But if certain recipes do not commend themselves to some of my readers, they are invited to remember that human palates differ considerably, and to try other dishes with the hope that they will like them better.

With the earnest desire that all who read this book will make some sincere endeavour to seek emancipation from the barbaric habits that are prevalent in Western lands, and to cease from that physical transgression in the matter of diet into which our forefathers, at some period of the world's history, appear to have fallen with such disastrous consequences to themselves and their posterity, it is sent forth upon its humble but beneficent mission. And I trust that many, when they have proved that such a way of living is both possible and advantageous, will strive to persuade others to live as Children of God, rather than as the beasts of prey.

Those who have reached that spiritual plane where the sacredness of all sentient life becomes recognised, and who find it painful to contemplate the wanton and cruel slaughter which at present takes place throughout Christendom—involving the death of at least a million large animals every day—must instinctively experience a longing to apprehend some way by which this butchery can be brought to an end. Such will be able to perceive the real significance of, and necessity for, the twentieth-century crusade against human carnivoracity—the Moloch idol of these modern days. They will also feel individually constrained to co-operate in the great work of bringing about this practical and beneficent Reformation, and of giving to mankind the blessings that will result from it.

As in the case of all previous editions of this book, any financial profit derived from its sale will be devoted to the exaltation of these humane and philanthropic ideals—hence its presentation to The Order of the Golden Age. My readers, therefore, who feel that its circulation will tend to lessen the sum total of human and sub-human suffering, are invited to assist in securing for it a large circulation, by lending or presenting copies to their friends, and making it widely known. And to attain this end, the sympathetic aid of journalists and other leaders of public thought will be especially appreciated.

Sidney H. Beard.

January,1913.

THE TRUE IDEAL IN DIET.

The physical structure of Man is declared by our most eminent biologists and anatomists to be that of a *frugivorous* (fruit-eating) animal. It is, therefore, our Creator's intention that we should subsist upon the various fruits of the earth—not upon the products of the shambles.[1]

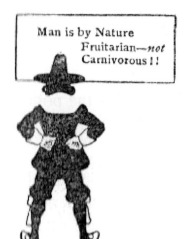

Man is by Nature Fruitarian—*not* Carnivorous!!

The accepted scientific classification places Man with the anthropoid apes, at the head of the highest order of mammals. These animals bear the closest resemblance to human beings, their teeth and internal organs being practically identical, and in a natural state they subsist upon nuts, seeds, grains, and other fruits. Hence those who have studied this subject thoroughly can hardly entertain any doubt that the more largely our diet consists of these simple products of nature, the more likely we shall be to enjoy health and to secure longevity.

The number and variety of such fruits and seeds is very great (including all the nuts and cereals *andtheirpr oducts*, as well as the pulses, legumes, etc.); and the Science of Dietetics has made such rapid progress in recent years that nuts and grains are, for the benefit of those who possess weakened digestive organs, now prepared in various ways which make them easily digestible and very savoury when cooked. To such foods may be added, for the sake of convenience and variety, vegetables of various kinds and dairy produce, such as milk, butter, cheese and eggs.

Personal Testimony. Nineteen years of abstinence from flesh-food (practised without any illness, and resulting in increased strength, stamina and health), and of observation and experiment during that period, combined with the knowledge obtained through helping hundreds of men and women to regain health by reforming their habits of living, have convinced me that a well selected fruitarian dietary, thus supplemented, will prove beneficial to all who desire physical and mental fitness. Temporary difficulties may be experienced by some in adopting such a simple style of living, or in obtaining adequate provision in their present domestic conditions; mistakes may be made—certain necessary elements being omitted from the new diet—and temporary failure may sometimes result in consequence; but if some preliminary study and consideration are given to the matter, and *variety* in the food is secured to ensure complete nourishment, success is easily obtainable.

A Step at a Time.

In most cases where there is a desire to adopt this purer and better way, it will be found that the policy of proceeding slowly but surely, a step at a time, is the wisest in the end.

The first step must be total abstinence from the flesh and blood of animals, and the substitution of less objectionable food containing an equal amount of proteid; this will soon lead to a distaste for fowl, but the use of fish should be retained by those commencing to reform their ways until some experience has been gained, and any serious domestic difficulties which may exist have been removed. Then this partial vegetarian diet can be still further purified, until it is more entirely "fruitarian" in its nature. Circumstances, and individual sentiment and taste, must regulate the rate of this progress towards what may be termed Edenic living; I can but show the way and give helpful information.

Advantages of Fruitarianism.

A few of the reasons which lead me to advocate a fruitarian dietary as the ideal one, are as follows:—

Persons who live chiefly upon fruits of all kinds do not injure themselves by consuming the poisonous waste-products (uric acid, &c.), contained in flesh; and they are not often tempted, like those who partake of very savoury and toothsome dishes, to eat after the needs of the body are satisfied. They thus escape two of the chief causes of disease and premature death—*auto-intoxication and excessive eating*. They also avoid, to a great extent, the temptation to eat when they are not hungry, and thus they are more likely to obey the dictates of natural instinct concerning *when to eat*. Even if fruit should be taken in excessive quantity, very little harm results from such indiscretion.

Fruitarians thus lessen the amount of work put upon the digestive organs, and consequently have more energy to expend upon mental or physical labour. The grape sugar contained in sweet fruits—such as dates, figs, raisins and bananas—is assimilated almost without effort and very quickly.

The juices of ripe fruits help to eliminate urates, waste products, and other harmful deposits from the blood and tissues, as they act as solvents. Fruit, therefore, tends to prevent ossification of the arteries, premature old age, gouty and rheumatic disorders, sickness and untimely death.

Fruitarian diet—if scientifically chosen and containing all the elements required by the body—prevents the development of the "drink crave," and it will cure nearly all cases if properly and wisely adopted. Dipsomania is induced by malnutrition, by eating stimulating food, such as flesh, or by eating to excess; a fruitarian drunkard has not yet, so far as I am aware, been discovered in this country.

Pure blood is secured by living upon such food, and consequently there is little or no tendency to develop *inflammatory* maladies. The wounds of Turkish and Egyptian soldiers have been found to heal three times as quickly as those of shamble-fed Englishmen; the reason is that they live chiefly upon dates, figs and other fruits, milk and lentils, etc.; and the same tendency has been observed in the case of the Japanese wounded. A wonderful immunity from sickness is enjoyed by those who live in accord with Nature's plan; microbes and disease germs do not find a congenial environment in their bodies. This I have proved by nearly twenty years of uninterrupted good health, and freedom from medical attendance, and my experience is corroborated by that of a multitude of witnesses in the ranks of the food-reformers.

Fruitarian diet, if complete, tends to lessen irritability, to promote benevolence and peace of mind, to increase the supremacy of the 'higher self,' to clear and strengthen spiritual perception, and to lessen domestic care. Those who desire to develop the higher spiritual powers which are latent in Man, to cultivate the psychic or intuitive senses, and to win their way to supremacy over their physical limitations, will find fruitarianism helpful in every respect. Such have only to *try it*, intelligently, in order to prove that this is true.

Such a system of living may thus become an important factor in the great work of uplifting our race from the *animal* to the *spiritual* plane; and herein lies the great hope for mankind. The harbingers of the 'Coming Race'—a more spiritual Race—are already treading this Earth, known and recognized by those whose eyes have been opened to the vision of the higher and transcendent life. And that which tends to accelerate the development of these characteristics is worthy of our serious consideration and earnest advocacy.

Such a diet does not necessitate the horrible cruelties of the cattle-boat and the slaughter-house—therefore it must commend itself to every genuine humanitarian.

It does not contain the germs of disease that are found in the dead bodies of animals—frequently afflicted with tuberculosis, cancer, foot-and-mouth-disease, incipient anthrax, swine-fever and parasites of various kinds.

It is free from that potent cause of physical malady, uric acid—which is contained in all flesh; and from "ptomaines,"—which develop in corpses quickly after death and often prove fatal to consumers of meat. And it will be found, if wisely chosen, to produce a stronger body, a clearer brain, and a purer mind.

The testimony of thousands of living advocates, both in cold and warm climates—many of whom are medical men, or athletes who have accomplished record performances which demanded prolonged endurance and unusual stamina—bears evidence to this fact; therefore those who are desirous of commencing this more excellent way of living need not fear they are making any reckless or dangerous experiment.

The food which our Creator *intended* us to eat must be the *safest* and *best* for us. Man does not resemble, either internally or externally, any carnivorous animal, and no unprejudiced student of the subject can well escape the conclusion that when we descend to the level of the beasts of prey, by eating flesh, we violate a physical Law of our being, and run the risk of incurring the inevitable penalties which Nature exacts for such transgressions.

These penalties are being lavishly dealt out with inexorable impartiality in the civilized lands of the Western world, where, in spite of the rapid

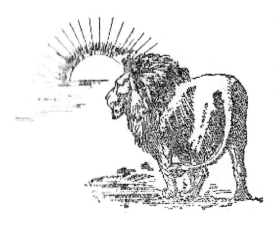

increase of our medical men, and the 'wonderful discoveries' of panaceas by the representatives of unscrupulous pathological search, such maladies as appendicitis, consumption, cancer, lunacy, gout, neurasthenia and other evidences of physical deterioration are still prevalent or steadily increasing.

And, although the fact is not so apparent to the superficial observer, a still heavier penalty in the form of spiritual loss is being suffered by those who err in this respect, for *carnalfood* produces *carnal-mindedness*, dims the spiritual vision, chains the soul to the material plane of thought and consciousness, and makes the supremacy of the 'spirit' over the 'flesh' well-nigh impossible.

It is natural for every man and woman to live at least a century. The fact that thousands have done so, proves that the majority might attain this age if they would cease from transgressing Nature's laws. Seneca truly said, "Man does not die, he kills himself."

By "eating to live," instead of "living to eat"—introducing into our bodies pure and vitalizing energy by means of wisely chosen natural food—and by amending our ways generally in accordance with the dictates of reason and common sense, we may live to benefit the world by useful service with our faculties matured and our minds stored by the teachings of experience. Instead of being in our dotage when we reach threescore years and ten, we should still be fit to serve our day and generation.

The Highest Motive.

Those who decide to adopt this reformed system of diet will be fortified in their resolve if they are actuated by loyalty to the Divine Will and regard for Humane Principle, in addition to reasons which are based merely upon self-interest. The desire to lessen suffering, and to live in accordance with God's laws, furnishes a stronger incentive than the wish to escape disease and to secure longevity.

A philanthropist or humanitarian who embraces the sublime ideal of helping to lift mankind to a higher plane of experience, to deliver our degenerate Race from some of the worst evils which afflict us, and, at the same time, to prevent the infliction of pain and death in most revolting forms upon countless millions of innocent animals, will either conquer the initial difficulties which confront those who thus make practical protest against the flesh traffic, or will cheerfully endure temporary inconvenience and self-denial "for Righteousness' sake."

Each new recruit who joins the Food-Reform Movement should therefore give such preliminary study to the subject as will produce the unalterable conviction that flesh-eating is an *unnatural* habit for Man, that it is totally *unnecessary*, that reliable medical evidence proves it to be generally *injurious*, and that it involves cruelty and bloodshed which are barbarous and indefensible, *becausequiteneedless* .

A deaf ear will then be turned to the warnings of any well-disposed friends who, being under the spell of ancient fallacies, or ignorant concerning the nutritive advantages which the fruits of the earth possess over the products of the shambles, would seek to deter him from the path of self-reform by prophesying physical shipwreck and disaster.

Popular illusions concerning the necessity for animal food are rapidly being swept away, and public opinion has already changed to such an extent that leaders of thought in every land are now impressed with the full import and beneficence of this Reformation. And so many forces are now converging and combining to influence and impel mankind in this direction, that the 'signs of the times' indicate a rapidly approaching Era in which Man will return to his original food, and, by so doing, enter upon a happier and more peaceful period of existence upon this planet.

1 See "The Testimony of Science in Favour of Natural and Humane Diet."

A PLEA FOR THE SIMPLE LIFE.

Simple meals and simple dishes are easily prepared, they lessen domestic care, are less likely to cause indigestion, and soon become appreciated and preferred.

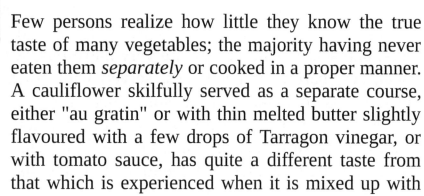

Few persons realize how little they know the true taste of many vegetables; the majority having never eaten them *separately* or cooked in a proper manner. A cauliflower skilfully served as a separate course, either "au gratin" or with thin melted butter slightly flavoured with a few drops of Tarragon vinegar, or with tomato sauce, has quite a different taste from that which is experienced when it is mixed up with gravy, meat, potatoes and other articles or food.

Young green peas, or new potatoes steamed in their skins and dried off in the oven so as to be "floury," will, if eaten with a little salt and butter, have a delicacy of flavour which is scarcely noticeable if they are served with a plate of beef or mutton and other vegetables. A few chestnuts carefully cooked in a similar manner, make a dish that an overfed alderman might enjoy; and the same remark will apply to many simple and easily prepared fruitarian dishes.

It is a mistake to think that this reformed diet necessarily involves a great amount of cooking, for the reverse is the fact if *simplicity* is aimed at and its advantages are appreciated. It is well to remember also that our most enlightened and progressive physicians are now recommending uncooked foods of all kinds to all who would retain or regain health.

An excellent lunch can be made with some well chosen cheese and brown bread and butter, and a delicate lettuce (dressed with pure olive oil, a small quantity of French wine vinegar, and a pinch of sugar), followed by fresh and dried fruits such as bananas, almonds, raisins, figs, etc. Such a repast is inexpensive, nutritious, and easily digestible. A large variety of foreign and fancy cheeses are now obtainable, so that even such a simple meal as this can be varied constantly. The best lettuces are produced by our French neighbours, but our own market gardeners are beginning to learn that it is easy to get them tender by growing them under glass.

The Simple Breakfast.

In most fruitarian households the cooking for breakfast soon becomes simplified and lessened. Eggs served in different ways on alternate mornings, fresh and dried fruits, nuts, brown bread, super cooked cereals such as granose biscuit, butter and preserves, are found to be quite sufficient as accompaniments to the morning beverage. French plums, figs and other dried fruits, when carefully stewed in the oven for some hours, and served with cream, are very nutritious. A small plate of 'Manhu' wheat, rye, barley, or oat flakes, served with hot milk or cream, can be added so as to make a more solid meal for growing children or hard workers. And those who are accustomed to a more elaborate breakfast, because of the difficulty of obtaining a mid-day substantial meal, can select one of the items which are mentioned in the list of recipes under the heading of "Breakfast Dishes."

Avoid Dyspepsia.

One reason for urging simplicity is that, owing to prevalent ignorance concerning food-values, it is more easy for the *inexperienced* food-reformer to make dietetic mistakes than the flesh-eater.

By partaking freely of stewed acid fruits and vegetables at the same meal, or by blending a great variety of savouries, vegetables, sweets and rich fatty dishes together in a ghastly 'pot pourri,' or by eating to excess of porridge, beans, or fried dishes, many have made serious blunders. They, for want of proper instruction, have hastily come to the conclusion that "vegetarian diet does not suit them," and returning to the flesh-pots, have henceforth denounced the evangel of dietetic reform, instead of profiting by the useful lesson Nature tried to teach them.

The wisest plan is to make one's diet generally *as varied as possible*, but not to mix many articles together *atthesamemeal* .

Abstainers from flesh should begin to live to some extent (say two days a week) in picnic style, and the practice will soon become more habitual. A picnic luncheon which is considered enjoyable in the woods or on the moors will be found to be just as nice at home if the articles provided are well chosen and tastefully prepared. Variety can be obtained by introducing daintily cut sandwiches made with mustard and cress, tomato paste, potted haricots, or lentils, scrambled eggs, fancy cheese cut thinly, flaked nuts and honey, etc. Fresh and dried fruit, nuts, almonds, raisins and sultanas, fruit cakes, and custard or rice puddings, provide useful additions; and it will soon be found that the old-fashioned three or four-course meal which involves such laborious preparation is a needless addition to life's many cares.

Necessary Elements in Food.

It is important to bear in mind that our daily food must contain a sufficient quantity of certain necessary elements:

(1) PROTEIN. To be found in nuts and nut foods (such as Protose, Nuttoria and Fibrose, &c.), eggs, cheese, brown bread, oatmeal, haricots, lentils and peas.

(2) FAT. To be obtained in nuts, nut-butters, olive oil, cheese, milk, cream, butter, and oatmeal.

(3) PHOSPHATES AND MINERAL SALTS. Contained in the husk of wheat, barley, oats, and rye (therefore included in brown bread, granose biscuits and other whole-wheat or cereal preparations), cheese, bananas and apples.

(4) SUGAR. To be obtained from all starch foods, but most easily and in the best and most readily assimilable form from sweet fruits and honey.

A PLEA FOR MODERATION.

One of the most frequent mistakes made by those who commence to live upon a fleshless diet is that of eating too much—an error, also committed 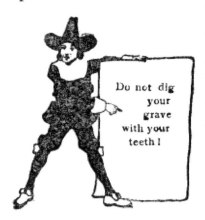 by the general public. Often, through ignorance of the fact that lean beef consists of water to the extent of about 75%, and through having been brought up under the spell of the popular delusion that meat is a great source of strength and stamina, they jump to the conclusion that they must consume large plates of cereals and vegetables in order to make up for their abstinence from animal food. They bring upon themselves severe attacks of dyspepsia—either by eating excessive quantities of starch in the form of porridge, bread and potatoes, or of such concentrated foods as haricots, lentils or nuts (being ignorant of the fact that these latter are much more nutritious than lean beef and that only a very small quantity is needed for a sufficient meal).[2]

Nothing does more injury to the Food-Reform Movement than the discredit which is brought upon it by those who upset themselves by over-eating, and who feel led to justify their defection by attacking the system they have forsaken. Among the numerous cases brought to my notice, I remember one of a minister's wife, who by partaking of seven meals a day, and finishing up at ten o'clock in the evening with cocoa, cheese and porridge, brought herself to such a state of nervous prostration that her local doctor ordered her to return to a flesh diet, "as she required *nourishment*." He thus diagnosed her condition, instead of attributing it to preposterous over-feeding.

A Golden Rule for every food-reformer is this—*Eat only when you are hungry,* and never to repletion. An exception must be made, however, in certain cases of anæmic and delicate persons. When there is not sufficient vitality to cause appetite, or to digest food normally, it is often necessary to insist on regular meals being taken, notwithstanding the patient's distaste for food. Drowsiness and stupor after a meal are sure signs of excess, and I cannot too strongly urge temperance in diet. During my long experience of philanthropic work as an advocate of natural and hygienic living, I have only heard of a few cases of persons suffering any ill effects from eating too little, whereas cases of the opposite sort have been rather numerous. Ninety-nine per cent. of the centenarians of the world have been characterized by *abstemiousness*; however much their ways and customs may have otherwise differed, in this one respect they are practically alike—declaring that they have always been small eaters, and believers in moderation in all things.

ARTISTIC COOKERY.

In every household where reformed diet is adopted, effort should be made to prepare the meals in an artistic manner. If a dish is skilfully cooked and tastefully served it is not only more enjoyable but more easily digested.

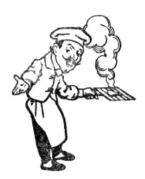

The general custom in English homes is to serve vegetables in a rather slovenly style. To see how nicely such things as legumes, vegetables, salads and fruits can be prepared, one requires to go to a good French or Italian restaurant. But it is quite easy for us to learn the ways of our friends abroad, and to make our dishes look tempting and appetising.

One of the first lessons to be learned by the vegetarian cook is how to fry rissoles, potatoes, etc., *quite crisp*, and free from any flavour of oil or fat. To do this a wire basket which will fit loosely into a stewpan is necessary, and it can be purchased at any good ironmonger's shop. Nutter (refined coconut butter) is a well prepared form of vegetable fat, and it is retailed at a moderate price; it keeps for a long period and is equally useful for making pastry—three quarters of a pound being equal to one pound of butter. Where nut-butters cannot be obtained, good olive oil should be used.

The temperature of the fat or oil must be past boiling point, and should reach about 380 degrees. When it is hot enough it will quickly turn a small piece of white bread quite brown, if a finger of it is dipped in the fat. Unless this temperature is reached the articles to be fried may turn out greasy and unbearable. If the fat is heated very much beyond 400 degrees it may take fire. Haricots, lentils, and many other legumes are more tasty if made into cutlets or rissoles and fried in this manner, after being mixed with breadcrumbs and seasoning, than if merely boiled or stewed in the usual crude style.

The Art of Flavouring.
The art of flavouring is also one which should be studied by every housewife. By making tasty gravies and sauces many a dish which would otherwise be insipid can be rendered attractive. The recipes for "Gravies" will prove useful on this point.

Many valuable modern scientific food products are not fully appreciated because people do not know how to serve them. Take 'Protose,' 'Nuttoria' and 'Nuttose' for instance—very useful substitutes for flesh which are made from nuts (malted and therefore half digested). If *slightly* stewed, and eaten without any flavouring, some persons dislike the distinctive taste; if, however, they are well cooked, according to the recipes printed later on in this book, and served with such garnishings as are recommended, they are usually much enjoyed, even by those who are prejudiced against all vegetarian ideas.

Cooking by Gas saves Labour.
Cooking by gas appliances is more easily controlled and regulated than when the old-fashioned fire is employed, and much labour for stoking and cleaning is avoided. Those who can do so, should obtain a gas hot-plate, consisting of two or three spiral burners, and a moderate-sized

gas oven. If they cannot afford the ordinary gas cooking oven, a smaller substitute can be obtained, which can be placed upon any gas jet; this is very economical for cooking single dishes, and for warming plates, etc. A gas cooking jet can be obtained for eighteenpence, and two or three of these will take the place of a hot-plate if economy is necessary. In summer-time the kitchen range is quite a superfluity unless it is required for heating bath water.

A New Mission for Women. The ordinary public know very little of the variety and delicacy of a well chosen fruitarian dietary when thoughtfully prepared; ignorance and prejudice consequently cause thousands to turn a deaf ear to the evangel of Food-Reform. All women who desire to bring about the abolition of Butchery, and to hasten the Humane Era, should therefore educate themselves in artistic fruitarian cookery, and then help to instruct others.

To illustrate the truth of these remarks I may mention that at a banquet given by the Arcadian Lodge of Freemasons, at the Hotel Cecil, in London—the first Masonic Lodge which passed a resolution to banish animal-flesh from all its banquets—one of the Chief Officers of the Grand Lodge of England attended. He came filled with prejudice against the innovation and prepared to criticise the repast most unfavourably. In his after-dinner speech, however, he admitted that it was one of the best Masonic banquets he had ever attended, and said that if what if he had enjoyed was "vegetarian diet," he was prepared to adopt it if he found it possible to get it provided at home.

By practising the recipes which are given in the following pages, and by utilizing the hints which accompany them, readers of this book will find no difficulty in acquiring the skill which is requisite to win many from the flesh-pots, even when they cannot be induced to abandon them from any higher motives than self-interest or gustatory enjoyment.

Every woman should resolve to learn how to feed her children with pure and harmless food. Every mother should make her daughters study this art and thus educate them to worthily fulfil their domestic responsibilities. Here is a new profession for women—for teachers of high-class fruitarian and hygienic cookery will soon be greatly in demand.

WHAT TO DO WHEN TRAVELLING.

The difficulty of being properly catered for when staying at Hotels was formerly a very real one, but owing to the enlightenment concerning diet which is now taking place, and the rapid 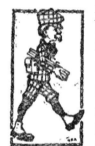 increase of foreign restaurants and cafés in English-speaking countries it is becoming lessened every day. The great variety of fleshless dishes now supplied in nearly all light-refreshment restaurants, in response to the public demand, is compelling even the largest Hotels to modify their cuisine accordingly.

For breakfast it is sometimes a good plan to order what one wants the previous night, if any specially cooked dishes are required, but it is *not* advisable to inform the waiter that one is a vegetarian. It is generally possible to obtain porridge, grilled tomatoes on toast, poached or fried eggs, stewed mushrooms, etc., without giving extra trouble or exciting comment. Where these cannot be obtained, a plain breakfast of brown bread or toast and butter, with eggs, preserves and fruit should be taken.

At large hotels in our chief cities a Restaurant and a Grill Room are provided. The food-reformer should go to one of these for his dinner, rather than to the dining room, as he will then be able to obtain various simple *à la carte* dishes. One 'portion' of any particular dish will often suffice for two persons, thus enabling those whose means are limited to obtain greater variety without increasing expenditure. Care has to be exercised, however, concerning certain dishes; for instance, if macaroni is required, it is well to ask the waiter to request the cook not to introduce any chopped ham. He should be told that you wish macaroni served with tomato sauce and cheese only, in the "Neapolitan" style.

In most Continental Hotels and Restaurants the simplest, cheapest, and best plan is to take 'table d'hôte'—telling the head waiter well beforehand that the lunch or dinner is required 'maigre' (that is without flesh, just as it is usually served during Lent). A varied, well selected, and ample repast will then be supplied at a moderate cost. The same plan is best in 'Pensions.'

The general rule to be adopted in small British hotels is to think beforehand what dishes the cook is in the habit of making which are free from flesh; these should be ordered in preference to those which are strange and not likely to be understood. At the same time it is well to insist upon being supplied with anything which it is reasonable to expect the proprietor to furnish, because such action tends to improve the catering of the hotels of the country, to make it easier for other food-reformers, and to sweep away the difficulty which at present exists in some towns, of obtaining anything fit to eat in the orthodox hotel coffee rooms, except beasts, birds, or fishes.

Railway Journeys. Those who are making railway journeys can easily provide themselves with a simple luncheon basket containing fruits, sandwiches made with flaked nuts, eggs, cheese or preserves, or with such delicacies as haricot or lentil potted meat (directions for making which will be found later on, in the section devoted to Luncheon Recipes.) Travellers may perhaps be reminded that cheese and nuts contain much more nutriment than lean meat.

Food-reformers who are about to pay a prolonged visit in a private house should inform the hostess, when accepting her invitation, that they are abstainers from flesh, but that their tastes are very simple and that they enjoy anything except flesh food. As she might have erroneous ideas about the requirements of vegetarians she might otherwise feel perplexed as to what to provide. If the visitor takes fish the fact should be stated.

No Faddism. Care should be taken not to involve the hostess in any needless trouble, and she should be shown, by the simplicity of one's requirements, that she is easily capable of affording complete satisfaction. When she realizes this, she will probably take pleasure in learning something about hygienic living, and will be ready to read a pamphlet or a guide-book upon the subject, and to produce some of the dishes contained in it.

The Humane Diet Cause has been much hindered by the 'fads' of persons who have adopted very extreme views about diet and who worry themselves and other people about trifling matters in connection with their food until they are almost regarded as being pests in a household. Instead of cheerfully partaking of anything that is provided, except flesh, they parade their scruples about almost everything on the table, and, consequently, those who entertain them vow that they will never become such nuisances themselves or entertain such again.

I have always found that by letting my friends clearly understand that I abstain from butchered flesh chiefly because of *humane reasons* and for the sake of *principle*, they respect my sentiment, and evince a desire to discuss the matter without prejudice. If fruitarianism is adopted merely as a 'fad,' discordant vibrations are often aroused because one's acquaintances consider that one is giving needless trouble by being unconventional without sufficient justification.

Sea Voyages. Those who are making a sea voyage will find that many of the large steamship companies are quite prepared to furnish substitutes for flesh-diet if an arrangement is made beforehand. In such cases there should be a clear stipulation that brown bread, dried and fresh fruit, nuts, farinaceous puddings, omelets, or dishes made with cheese, macaroni, lentils, haricots, tomatoes, etc., should be obtainable in some form and in sufficient variety. A list of a few 'specialities' (such as Protose, Nuttoria, &c.) should be furnished when a long voyage is contemplated, so that the steward may stock them.

ADVICE FOR BEGINNERS.

The following suggestions will prove helpful to those who are desirous of adopting the reformed dietary:—

1. Give up flesh meat *at once* and *entirely*—replacing it by dishes made with eggs, cheese, macaroni, peas, lentils, nuts, and nut-meats. Later on you will be able to do without fish also, but it is best to proceed slowly and surely.

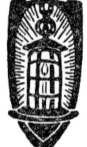

2. Eat *less* rather than *more*. Fruitarian foods such as the above are more nourishing than butcher's meat.

3. Try to like *simple* foods, instead of elaborate dishes that require much preparation. Avoid 'frying-panitis.'

4. Eat dry foods rather than sloppy ones; they are more easily digested. Take toast or Granose biscuits with porridge to assist proper salivation. If porridge causes trouble, use wheat or rye flakes (Manhu or Kellogg brands), with hot milk or cream, instead.

5. Do not mix stewed acid fruits with vegetables and legumes; take the former with cereals, cheese, or eggs. Green vegetables should be taken very sparingly, and with savoury dishes alone. If eaten with sweets they are apt to disagree.

6. Persons of sedentary habits should let at least one meal a day consist of uncooked fruit only —or of fruit with brown bread and butter—the bread being *well baked*.

7. Dried fruits, such as figs, dates, prunes, raisins, sultanas, etc., are very easily digested; and if blended with nuts or almonds they make a perfect meal. Such fruits may be taken freely and with advantage by almost everyone.

8. Nuts should be flaked in a nut-mill to aid digestion; cheese can also be made more easily assimilable in this way (or by cooking). Many nut products are now sold which are malted and partially pre-digested.

9. Give a few hours' thought and study to the important subject of your diet; learn what to do, and what newly-invented scientific foods are obtainable.

10. Do not make the mistake of attempting to live on potatoes, white bread, cabbages, etc., or merely upon the ordinary conventional dietary with the meat left out. Obtain and use well made and well cooked wholemeal bread every day. Take sufficient *proteid*, 1½ to 2-ozs. per day, to avoid anæmia—indigestion often results from *lack of vitality* caused through chronic semi-starvation.

11. If you feel any symptoms of dyspepsia, and can trace it to *excess* in eating, or to dietetic errors, reduce your food, fast temporarily, and take more exercise. Consider what mistakes you have made, and avoid them in the future. Eat only when hungry, in such cases.

Commercial Dietetic Inventions.

A large number of special proprietary substitutes for animal food can now be obtained to supplement the ordinary ones provided in the household. The latest particulars concerning these can always be known by reference to the advertisement pages of *The Herald of the Golden Age*, and full information as to their use is supplied by the various manufacturers. But although they are *useful* and *convenient* in many households, they are not *absolutely essential*. 'Home-made' dishes are often the best, being most economical, therefore it is advisable that all food-reformers should learn how to make nut-meats, &c., at home. Some of these substitutes are as follows:—

For Meat-Extracts: Marmite, Vegeton, Carnos, Nutril, Mapleton's Gravy Essence, Cayler's Extract, Wintox.

For Joints of Meat: Protose, Nuttose, Savrose, Fibrose, F.R. Nut-Meat, Vejola, Nuttoria, Shearn's Nut-Meat, Nutton, Brazose, Nuto-Cream Meat, Mapleton's Frittamix.

For Cold Meats: "Pitman" Nut-Meat Brawn, Ellis's Tomato and Nut Paste, Pasta-sol, Lentose, Nuska Viando, Savoury Paste, Potted Beans and Lentils.

For Meat Fat: Nutter Suet, Vegsu, Nutter, Nucoline, and Nut Margarine.

Pine Kernels, which contain 10 ozs. of oil to the pound, and which when rolled and chopped exactly resemble suet, are also an excellent substitute.

Delicious Nut-Butters are also now obtainable for high-class cookery—such as Almond, Walnut, Cashew, and Table Nutter. Although superior, these are as cheap as ordinary cooking butters.

For Lard and Dripping: Nutter, Darlene, Albene, Nut-oil, "Pitman" Vegetable Lard.

For Meat proteid: Emprote, Hygiama, Horlick's Malted Milk, Casumen Dried Milk, Gluten Meal.

For Gelatine: Agar-Agar, or Cayler's Jellies.

For Animal Soups: Mapleton's Nut and proteid Soups, and "Pitman" Vegsal Soups.

Prepared Breakfast Cereals: Manhu flaked Wheat, Rye, Barley and Oats, Kellogg Wheat and Corn Flakes, Granose Flakes and Biscuits, Shredded Wheat, Archeva Rusks, Puffed Wheat, Power, Kornules, Toasted Wheat Flakes, Melarvi Crisps and Biscuits.

For Picnic Hampers: Savage's Nut Foods or Cream o' Nuts, Wallace Cakes and Scones, Mapleton's Nut Meats, Winter's Nut Cream Rolls, "Pitman" Fruit and Nut Cakes and Nut Meat Brawn, Wallace P. R. or Ixion or Artox or "Pitman" Biscuits.

Meat Stock is substituted by vegetable stock, produced by stewing haricots, peas, lentils, etc. The latter is far more nutritious, and is free from the uric acid and excrementitious matter that are present in meat decoctions. A tasty and meaty flavour can be at once given to soups or gravies by adding some vegetable meat-extract selected from one of the varieties already mentioned.

In the following pages recipes will be found for preparing dishes which closely resemble, in taste, appearance, and nutritive value, those to which the community have been accustomed, some of them being of such a nature that persons who are fond of flesh-food find it difficult to detect whether they are eating such or not.

RELATIVE VALUES OF FOODS.

How to Regulate our Diet.

Our food must contain certain elements, and in proper quantity, if the body is to be well sustained, renewed and nourished. These are mainly as follows:

1. Protein to form flesh, build muscle, and produce strength.

2. Fat and Carbohydrates, to provide heat and energy.

3. Salts and minerals (such as phosphates, lime, iron, citrates, etc.) to build bones and teeth, feed the brain and nerves, and purify the body.

No hard-and-fast table or rule can be laid down concerning the proper proportions in which these elements should be combined, because the amount needful for each individual varies according to his size, the sort of work he does, the amount of physical or mental energy he puts forth, and the temperature of the atmosphere surrounding him.

Until Professor Chittenden made his extensive and conclusive series of experiments in America, in 1903-4, to determine the real amount of Protein and other elements required to keep the body in perfect health, the average estimate for a person of average size, who does a moderate amount of physical labour, was about 4-ozs. of Protein per day.

But these official experiments, conducted with scientific precision, extending over a long period, and made with thirty-four typical and carefully graded representatives of physical and mental work, demonstrated that half this amount of Protein is sufficient, and that strength and health are increased when the quantity is thus reduced; also that a smaller amount of Carbohydrate food (bread, etc.), than was previously thought necessary, is enough.

One may therefore now safely reckon that men of average size and weight (say 10 to 12 stone) doing a moderate amount of physical and mental work, can thrive under ordinary circumstances on a daily ration containing about 800 grains of Protein (nearly 2 ozs).

The following food chart will enable the reader to calculate (approximately) how much food of any particular kind is necessary to provide the above amount. Adult persons below the average size and weight, and living sedentary rather than an active physical life, will naturally require less than this normal standard. The relative cost and economy of the different foods can also thus be ascertained.

If care is taken to secure a sufficient quantity of Protein the requisite amount of Carbohydrates is not likely to be omitted, and hunger will prove a reliable guide in most cases. It is advisable, however, to see that enough Fat is taken, especially in winter, and by persons lacking in nerve force.

The table of food-values will easily enable the reader to ascertain the proportion of Fat in each kind of food.

The following indications of dietetic error may prove useful:—

Signs of Dietetic Mistakes. Excess of proteid matter causes a general sense of plethora and unbearableness, nervous prostration or drowsiness after meals, a tendency to congestion (often resulting in piles, etc.), headache, irritability, and bad temper. A continuous deficiency of it would tend to produce general weakness and anæmia.

Excess of carbohydrate matter (starch), especially if not sufficiently cooked and not well masticated, produces dyspepsia, flatulence, pain in the chest and abdomen, acidity (resulting in pimples and boils), and an inflammatory state of the system. Deficiency of it (or its equivalent, grape sugar) would produce lack of force and physical exhaustion.

Excess of fat tends to cause biliousness. Deficiency of it results in nervous weakness, neuralgia, and low temperature of the body.

Food for Brain Workers. It is important to remember that the more *physical* energy we put forth, the larger is the amount of proteid we require in our diet—and vice versa. Brain workers of sedentary habits require but little proteid, and quickly suffer from indigestion if this is taken too freely. For such, a very simple dietary consisting largely of dried and fresh fruits, nuts (flaked or ground), milk, eggs and cheese, and *super-cooked* cereals (such as wholemeal biscuits, and toast, Granose and Kellogg flakes, and well baked rice dishes) will be found to be the most suitable.

In order to supply the brain with phosphates it is very important that mental workers should take whole wheat bread instead of the emasculated white substitute which is provided almost everywhere. It is the outer part of the grain that provides brain-food (combined with an *easily assimilable* form of protein), and many of our urban bread winners break down because they are deprived of the essential food elements therein contained. To take 'standard' bread does not meet the case, and every food-reformer who wants to keep really fit should demand and obtain well baked and unadulterated wholemeal bread. I feel convinced that if every growing child and every mental toiler could always be supplied with bread of this type, the deterioration of our British race would soon be arrested and we should witness signs of physical regeneration. 'Artox' and 'Ixion' brands of pure whole wheatmeal are the most perfect I know of at the present time, and delicious bread can easily be made from them if the recipe printed on page <u>114</u> is followed.

FOOD CHART.

Showing how to obtain sufficient (1) Protein—for body building. (2) Carbohydrates and Fat—for providing heat and energy.

A man of average size and weight (10 to 12 stone) doing a moderate amount of physical labour requires about 800 grains of Protein per day (nearly 2 ozs.). Women and sedentary workers require about 1½ ozs. (655 grains), and hard physical labourers about 1000 grains.

	Amount.	Grains of Protein.	Grains of Carbo-hydrates and Fat	Approximate Cost.	
				s.	d.
Protose (Nut meat)	8 ozs.	889	593		6
Fibrose (Nut meat)	12 ozs.	767	4015		9
Granose (Wheat)	13 ozs.	795	4424		9
Emprote (Eustace Miles Proteid Food)	6 ozs.	918	1320		7
Nuto-Cream	10 ozs.	870	3145		8
Manhu Flaked Wheat	13 ozs.	722	3935		3
Horlick's Malted Milk	7 ozs.	797	2548	1	6
Almonds	8 ozs.	805	2100		10
Chestnuts	13 ozs.	830	3700		3
Lentils	8 ozs.	900	1915		1½
Peas	8 ozs.	830	2100		1½
Haricots	8 ozs.	900	2030		2
Oatmeal	12 ozs.	813	3670		2
Cheese (Cheddar)	6 ozs.	745	823		3
"	6 ozs.	835	730		4
(Gruyère)	4 ozs.	770	262		3
"					

(Parmesan)					
"	5 ozs.	840	450		3
(Dutch)					
Bread (Artox Wholemeal)	24 ozs.	788	4524		3
Rice (once milled)	14 ozs.	810	2500		3
Eggs	7	856	640		7
Figs or Dates	2 lbs.	850	9100		10
Milk	3 pts.	859	1927		6
Milk (Skimmed)	3 pts.	800	742		3
For Comparison:—					
Lean Beef	10 ozs.	846	151		9
Mutton	13 ozs.	822	1107		10
Chicken	9 ozs.	850	185	1	9
Fish (Sole)	16 ozs.	824		1	3
"	12 ozs.	840	274	1	6
(Salmon)					

TABLE OF FOOD VALUES.

Compiled from such authorities as Church, Payer, Letheby, Blyth, Hemmeter, Pavy, Holbrook, Oldfield, Miles, and Broadbent, etc.

		PERCENTAGE OF					
		Water.	Protein.	Fat.	Starch Matter or Sugar.	Mineral Matter.	Total Nutriment.
FLESH-FOODS.	Lean Beef	72·0	19·3	3·6		5·1	28·0
	Veal	71·0	17·0	11·0		1·0	29·0
	Mutton(Medium Fat)	65·2	14·5	19·5		0·8	34·8
	Fat Pork	39·0	9·8	48·9		2·3	61·0
	Chicken (flesh)	72·4	21·6	4·7		1·3	27·6
	Fish (Sole)	86·1	11·9	0·2		1·2	13·3
	Salmon	77·0	16·1	5·3		1·5	23·0
EGGS.	Eggs.	64·0	14·0	10·5		1·5	26·0
	White of Egg	78·0	12·4			1·6	14·0
	Yolk of Egg	52·0	16·0	30·7		1·3	48·0
MILK AND MILK PRODUCTS.	Milk (Cow's)	86·0	4·1	3·9	5·2	0·8	14·0
	Cheese: Cheddar	36·0	28·4	31·1		4·5	64·0
	Stilton	32·0	26·2	37·8		4·0	67·0
	Gruyère	40·0	31·5	24·0		3·0	58·5
	Dutch	36·10	29·43	27·54			56·97
	Parmesan	27·56	44·08	15·95		5·72	65·75
	Butter	12·6		86·4		0·8	87·2

CEREALS AND FARINACEOUS FOODS.	Wheatmeal (Artox)	13·13	12·84	2·30	68·0	1·33	84·47
	Oatmeal	10·4	15·6	6·11	63·6	3·0	89·1
	Barley Meal	14·6	6·7	1·3	75·5	1·1	84·6
	Bran	12·5	16·4	3·5	43·6	6·0	69·5
	Rice (once milled)	10·4	11·4	0·4	79·0	0·4	91·2
	Macaroni (Best)	10·8	11·7	1·6	72·9	3·0	89·2
	Sago, Tapioca and Arrowroot	14·0	1·6	0·6	83·0	0·4	85·6
BREAD FOODS.	Wholemeal Bread (Artox)	46·0	7·5	1·4	42·0	1·3	52·2
	White Bread	40·0	3·5	1·0	51·2	1·0	56·5
	Granose Biscuits	3·1	14·2	1·7	77·5	1·9	95·3
LEGUMES.	Haricots (White)	9·9	25·5	2·8	55·7	3·2	87·2
	Lentils, Egyptian	12·3	25·9	1·9	53·0	3·0	83·0
	Peas (Dried)	8·3	23·8	2·1	58·7	2·1	86·7
	Peas (Green)	81·8	3·4	0·4	13·7	0·7	18·2
	Pea Nuts	6·5	28·3	46·2	1·8	3·3	79·6
NUTS.	Chestnuts	7·3	14·6	2·4	69·0	3·3	89·3
	Walnuts	7·2	15·8	57·4	13·0	2·0	88·2
	Filberts	38·0	18·4	28·5	11·1	1·5	59·5
	Brazil Nuts	6·0	16·4	64·7	6·6	3·3	91·0
	Coconuts	46·6	5·5	36·0	8·1	1·0	50·5
	Pine Kernels	5·0	9·2	70·5	14·0	0·3	94·0
	Almonds	6·2	23·5	53·0	7·8	3·0	87·3
FRESH FRUITS.	Bananas	74·1	1·9	0·8	22·9	1·0	26·6
	Apples	84·8	0·4	0·5	12·0	0·5	13·4
	Grapes	78·2	1·3	1·7	14·7	0·5	18·2
	Strawberries	87·6	1·1	0·7	6·8	0·6	9·2
DRIED FRUITS.	Raisins	14·0	2·5	4·7	64·7	4·1	76·0
	Figs	17·5	6·1	0·9	65·9	2·3	75·2
	French Plums	26·4	2·4	0·8	65·5	1·7	70·4
	Dates	20·8	6·6	0·2	65·3	1·6	73·7
VEGETABLES.	Carrots	86·5	1·2	0·3	9·2	0·9	11·6
	Turnips	90·3	0·9	0·15	5·0	0·8	6·85
	Cauliflower (Head)	90·8	2·2	0·4	4·7	0·8	8·1

Potatoes	75·0	2·2	0·2	21·0	1·0	24·4
Mushrooms	90·3	4·3	0·3	3·7	1·4	9·7
Tomatoes	91·9	1·3	0·2	5·0	0·7	7·2
Asparagus	93·7	1·8		0·7	0·5	3·0
Beet	87·5	1·3		9·0	1·1	11·4
Parsnip	82·0	1·2		0·6	7·2	9·0
Spinach	88·5	3·5		4·4	2·0	9·9
Cabbage	90·0	1·9		2·5	1·2	5·6

VEGETARIAN SOUPS.

VEGETABLE STOCK.

The best stock for vegetable soups is made from haricot beans. Take a pound of these, pick and wash well, and soak for 10 or 12 hours in cold water. Put them in a saucepan with the water in which they were soaked, add a few of the coarser stalks of celery, 1 or 2 chopped Spanish onions, a blade of mace, and a few white peppercorns. If celery is not in season, use celery salt. Bring to a boil, skim, and cook gently for at least 2 hours. Then strain, and use as required.

1. Artichoke Soup.

Take 2-lbs. of white artichokes, 3-pts. of water, 3 large onions, a piece of celery (or some celery salt), ¼-pt. of raw cream or 1-pt. of milk. Boil together for 45 minutes, strain through a fine sieve and serve. If cream is used it should not be added until after the soup is cooked.

2. Chestnut Soup.

Take 1-lb. chestnuts, 1 or 2 onions, 1½-pints vegetable stock, 1-oz. nut-butter.

Boil the chestnuts for 15 minutes and peel them; put these with the onions (sliced) into a roomy stewpan, with the butter, and fry briskly for 5 minutes; now add the stock, with seasoning to taste, and bring to the boil. Simmer gently until onions and chestnuts are quite soft, and pass all through a hair sieve. Dilute with milk until the consistency of thin cream, and serve with *croûtons*.

3. Rich Gravy Soup.

To 3-pts. of haricot stock add 1 onion and 1 carrot (fried with butter until brown), 1 stick of celery, 2 turnips and 6 peppercorns, and thicken with cornflour. Boil all together for 1 hour, strain, return to saucepan, and add 3 small teaspoons of Marmite. Warm it up, but *not to boiling point*. Serve with fried bread dice. This soup, if well made, is equal to anything that a French chef can produce.

4. Mock Turtle Soup.

Fry 6 good-sized onions in 1-oz. of butter till nicely browned, then add 2 breakfastcups of German lentils, a good handful of spinach leaves, a few capers, about 6 chillies, and 3 pints of water. Let this simmer for 2 or 3 hours, then strain off, add 2 tablespoons of tapioca which has been soaked for an hour or two. Boil till perfectly clear. When ready for serving add salt to taste and 1 teaspoonful of Nutril. Some small custard quenelles should be put in the tureen— made by beating 1 egg in 2-ozs. flour and adding ¼-pt. milk. Bake until firm and cut into dice.

5. Brown Haricot Soup.

oil ½-lb. beans in 2-qts. of water. When the beans crack, add a few tomatoes, 1 leek sliced, or a Spanish onion, and a bunch of herbs. Boil until the vegetables are tender, adding a little more water if necessary. Rub all through a sieve, and return to pan, adding seasoning, a good lump of butter, and the juice of half a small lemon after the soup has boiled. If a richer soup is required add two teaspoonfuls of Nuto-Cream or Marmite just before serving.

6. Tomato Soup.

Take a pound of tomatoes, a sliced onion, and 2-ozs. of tapioca (previously soaked for some hours). Boil for an hour, then add salt, pepper, and a little butter. Mix ½-pt. of milk with a teaspoonful of flour; add this to the soup, stir and boil for 5 minutes.

7. Egyptian Lentil Soup.

Wash and pick ½-lb. Egyptian lentils and put on to boil in about 1-qt. of water. Add 1 sliced onion, 1 carrot, 1 turnip, a small bunch of herbs, and celery salt, and boil gently about 1 hour. Rub through a sieve, return to pan, add 1-oz. butter and a cupful of milk. Bring to boil and serve.

8. Brazil Nut Soup.

Pass 1 pint of shelled Brazil nuts through a nut mill, fry these with one or two chopped onions in 1-oz. of nut-butter, keeping them a pale yellow colour; add 1-oz. flour, and gradually 1½-pts. of white stock; bring slowly to the boil and simmer gently until the onions are soft. Pass through a hair sieve, and dilute with milk.

9. Julienne Soup.

Cut some carrots, turnips, onions, celery, and leeks into thin strips, using double quantity of carrots and turnips. Dry them and then fry slowly in 2-ozs. of butter until brown. Add 2-qts. of clear vegetable stock and simmer until tender. Season with salt and a teaspoonful of castor sugar. Chop some chervil or parsley finely, add and serve. The addition of some green peas is an improvement—and also quenelles (see 4).

10. Green Lentil Soup.

Fry 5 onions in a large saucepan until brown. Add ¾-lb. of green lentils, 1-qt. water, and 2 sticks of celery. Stew for 2 hours, and pass through a strainer. Add ¼-lb. of cream and ½-pt. of milk, bring to the boil, flavour with salt, and serve.

11. White Soubise Soup.

(A French Recipe).

Take 2-ozs. butter, 4 good-sized onions, about 1-pt. cauliflower water, and 1-pt. of milk, sufficient bread (no crust) to very nearly absorb the liquor. Cut up the onions, put into the saucepan with the butter, and cook slowly till tender—it must not be brown. Now add the bread, the cauliflower water, and half the milk, and boil slowly for an hour. Take it off the fire, pass it through a sieve, add the rest of the milk, and heat it again, taking care it does not actually boil, as it may curdle. Serve.

12. Green Pea Soup.

One quart shelled peas; 3 pints water; 1 quart milk; 1 onion; 2 tablespoonfuls butter; 1 tablespoonful flour. Salt and pepper to taste.

Put the peas in a stewpan with the boiling water and onion and cook until tender (about half an hour). Pour off water, saving for use later. Mash peas fine, add water in which they were boiled, and rub through *purée* sieve. Return to saucepan, add flour and butter, beaten together, and the salt and pepper. Gradually add milk, which must be boiling hot. Beat well and cook 10 minutes, stirring frequently. This recipe is useful when green peas are getting old and are not tender enough to be enjoyable if served in the usual way.

13. White Haricot Soup.

Stew ½-lb. of beans in 2-qts. of water, adding 5 chopped onions, some chopped celery and a carrot which have been fried in some butter until well cooked; stew until the beans are tender, and strain if clear soup is required, or pass through a sieve for thick soup; add some cream and milk, bring to the boil, flavour with salt, and serve.

14. Marmite Vegetarian Soup.

Take a dessertspoonful of Marmite, 1-pt. of water or vegetable stock, a tablespoonful of fine sago or tapioca, a slice or two of any vegetables, with a sprig of parsley and a little salt. Boil the vegetables for a few minutes in the water, skim well, add the sago or tapioca, and boil for an hour or over, then strain; stir the Marmite in and serve hot. A delicious and cheap soup. A gill of milk or cream boiled and added at the end—omit the same measure of water—is an improvement in some cases.

15. Almond Soup.

(A nice Summer Soup).

One pint of white stock, 1 pint milk, 1 small breakfastcup of ground almonds, 1-oz. butter, 3-ozs. minced onions, 1-oz. flour. Fry the onion in the butter in a stewpan till a pale yellow colour, stir in the flour, and when well blended, moisten with some of the stock, adding the almonds, broth and milk by degrees till all are exhausted, bring to the boil, skim, and simmer *gently* for half an hour, pass through a hair sieve. Serve with nicely cooked green peas.

16. Celery Soup.

Six heads of celery, 1 teaspoon of salt, a little nutmeg, 1 lump sugar, 1 gill of stock, ½-pint of milk, and two quarts of boiling water.

Cut the celery into small pieces and throw it into the boiling water seasoned with nutmeg, salt and sugar, boil until sufficiently tender, pass it through a sieve, add the stock, and simmer for half-an-hour, then add the milk, bring it up to the boil and serve.

17. Potato Soup.

Four middle sized potatoes, a thick slice of bread, 3 leeks peeled and cut into slices, a teacup of rice, salt and pepper to taste, 2 qts. of water.

Bring the water up to boil, then put in all the ingredients except the rice, pepper and salt, cover and let them come to a brisk boil, add the rice and boil slowly for one hour.

18. Pea Soup.

Take 1½ pints of split peas and 3 onions. Put the peas to soak overnight, then cook with the onions until quite soft—pass through a sieve, add 1 gill of milk, bring to the boil. Serve with squares of fried bread or toast. Celery, salt, pepper and chopped mint may be added to taste.

19. Mock Hare Soup.

Soak some haricot beans over night in boiling water, then stew them for 2 hours in water with 2 onions, salt and pepper. When quite tender pass them through the sieve, add 1-oz. ground walnuts, boil again for 5 minutes, add forced meat balls, and serve.

20. Carrot Soup.

Two lbs. carrots, 3-ozs. butter, seasoning to taste, 2 quarts of bean stock or water.

Scrape the carrots, wash and wipe them quite dry, and cut in thick slices; put the butter in a large stewpan and when melted put the carrots in and stew gently for one hour without browning, then add the stock or water and simmer until tender (about an hour). Pass them through the sieve, add the seasoning and boil for 5 minutes; skim well and serve.

21. Onion Soup.

Put about 2 doz. small onions in a stewpan with 1-oz. butter, cover and let them stew for about 20 minutes, then add sufficient boiling water to cover them, boil till quite tender, pass through a sieve, boil up again, add the savoury seasoning and 1 gill of milk. A little boiled macaroni chopped up fine may be added before serving.

22. Carnos Soup.

Two tablespoons of Carnos in a pint of boiling water makes a very nourishing soup; it may be thickened with rice, vermicelli, spaghetti, etc., if required, and served with fingers of toast.

23. White Windsor Soup.

Take 4 breakfastcups of white stock, then add 6 tablespoons of mashed potatoes, and 1-oz. of sago. Stir over the fire till clear, then add 1 breakfastcupful of milk, and a little minced parsley. Let it come to boiling point, but no more. Serve in a very hot tureen.

SUBSTITUTES FOR FISH.

24. Mock Scallop Oysters.

Scrape some salsify roots, boil them until tender, drain. Beat with wooden spoon to a *smooth* paste free of *fibre*. Moisten with cream, add a teaspoonful of butter or a thick white sauce. Serve in fireproof china, or in scallop shells. Put breadcrumbs on top, which have been steeped in butter and browned.

25. Mock Oyster Patties.

Make the above mixture, put it into short puff paste made into patties, and bake until a nice brown tint.

26. Green Artichokes.

(A substitute for Oysters).

Boil some green artichoke heads until tender (about 1 hour) and serve hot. Mix some French wine vinegar and pure olive oil (one teaspoonful of vinegar to three of oil) with a pinch of salt and pepper.

Strip off the leaves one by one and dip the fleshy ends in the dressing; then scrape off the tender part of the leaf with the teeth. When the leaves are stripped, cut out the centre of the 'crown' and cut off its stalk quite short. Remove the seeds, and the crown itself will then be found a bonne bouche.

27. Fried Chinese Artichokes.

Boil the artichokes until tender. After draining, drop them into batter of fine breadcrumbs and egg. Fry crisp and serve with parsley sauce and slices of lemon.

28. Mock Fish Cutlets.

Two ozs. rice, 4-ozs. white haricot beans, ½-gill of thick curry sauce, pepper and salt, egg and breadcrumbs.

Make a thick curry sauce, add to it the boiled rice and beans chopped up fine, pepper and salt. Cook together for a few minutes, then turn out on a plate and leave to cool. Form into balls or small flat cakes, dip in egg, then crumbs, and fry in boiling oil.

29. Fillets of Mock Sole.

Bring to a boil half a pint of milk, and stir in 2-ozs. of ground rice. Add 1-oz. of butter, a teaspoonful of grated onion, and a pinch of mace; also 3 large tablespoonfuls of potato which has been put through a fine sieve. Mix and let all simmer slowly in the saucepan for 15 minutes. The mixture should be fairly stiff. When removed from the fire, add 1 egg and 1 yolk well beaten. Mix thoroughly, and turn out on a flat dish not quite half an inch thick, and allow it to get quite cold. Then divide into fillet-shaped pieces, brush over with the beaten white of egg, toss in fine breadcrumbs, and fry in plenty of smoking-hot fat. Drain, and serve very hot, garnished with slices of lemon, and with Hollandaise sauce.

30. Mock Fish Roe.

Peel and slice 3 or 4 tomatoes, and put in a saucepan with nearly half a pint of water, and some grated onion. Cook until the tomato is soft and smooth; then sprinkle in sufficient maize meal to make the mixture fairly stiff, add pepper and salt and one heaped tablespoonful of grated cheese. Form into fillets or cutlets, and fry in the usual way.

31. Filleted Salsify.

Cook some salsify until tender, slice it into quarters lengthways, and cut it into 3-in. lengths; dip in egg and breadcrumbs, and fry crisp; serve with parsley sauce (recipe 164), and garnish with slices of lemon and parsley.

32. Mock White Fish.

Boil ½-pt. milk and thicken with rather more than 1-oz. of semolina, to make a little stiffer than for rice mould. Add a lump of butter, salt, a little grated onion and a saltspoonful of mace, and let all cook together for 10 minutes, stirring frequently. Boil 3 potatoes and put through masher, and whilst hot add to the semolina or it will not set well. Pour into dish to stiffen, and when quite cold cut into slices, roll in egg and white breadcrumbs, fry crisp in Nutter and serve with parsley sauce as a fish course. The mixture must be stiff, for the frying softens the semolina again.

33. Mock Hake Steaks.

Put in a pan 3-ozs. breadcrumbs, with ½-pint of milk and a pinch of salt. Stir over a slow fire for a few minutes; then add 2-ozs. flour, the yolk of 1 egg, 3-ozs. grated cheese, 1-oz. butter, and a pinch of mace. Cook for fifteen minutes; when quite cold form into fritters, dip in egg and breadcrumbs, and fry in boiling oil till a nice golden brown. Serve with piquante sauce.

SUBSTITUTES FOR MEAT DISHES.

34. Walnut Cutlets.

Put a small cap of milk and ½-oz. of butter in a saucepan on the fire. When it boils add 3-ozs. of *dried* and *browned* breadcrumbs and a little dredging of flour. Let it cook until it no longer adheres to the pan, and remove from the fire. When it is cool add 2 eggs, beating until smooth, a large tablespoonful of shelled walnuts (previously run through the nut mill), seasoning, and a little grated onion juice. Mix well and shape into cakes about ½-in. thick on a floured board. Roll in flour or egg and breadcrumbs, and fry. Serve with walnut gravy, or round a dish of grilled tomatoes.

35. Brown Bean Cutlets.

Boil one pint of brown haricot beans until soft, strain and keep the stock; pass the beans through a sieve and add a tablespoonful of chopped parsley, a little grated onion, pepper, salt, a small piece of butter, and, if liked, a few drops of A1 Sauce. Add breadcrumbs until the right consistency is obtained for moulding into cutlet form. Egg, crumb, and fry as usual. Serve with tomato sauce or a rich gravy.

36. Green Pea Cutlets.

Green pea cutlets, either fresh or dried, may be made the same way as stated in the previous recipe, substituting a little chopped mint for the parsley and onion, and serving with mint sauce, and a nice brown gravy made from the green pea stock.

37. Haricot Cutlets.

Boil 1-pt. of brown or white haricot beans with one or two onions till quite soft, strain and pass through a sieve, add some chopped parsley, a tablespoonful of grated pine kernels, a little tapioca (previously soaked in cold water), pepper and salt and a few breadcrumbs. Mould into cutlets, egg, crumb, and fry. Serve with sliced lemon and parsley sauce, or with brown gravy.

38. Walnut Rissoles.

Take ½-pt. ground walnuts, ½-pt. breadcrumbs, 1-oz. butter, 1-oz. flour, a little milk, chopped parsley, and pepper and salt to taste. Make a thick white sauce with butter, flour and milk, add all the other ingredients. Mix well and form into rissoles, dip in egg, then in crumbs, and fry crisp in boiling oil. These may be glazed and eaten cold with a salad and mint sauce.

39. Stuffed Vegetable Marrow.

Peel a medium sized marrow, and remove the seeds, keeping the marrow whole. Prepare the following stuffing:—

Mix 2 or 3 chopped and fried onions, 6-ozs. pine kernels (these should be ground and also fried with the onions), 6-ozs. breadcrumbs, pepper and salt, 1 chopped hard boiled egg, and 1 raw egg to bind. Fill the marrow with this mixture, and steam for half an hour to partly cook the marrow. Now place in a baking tin, cover with breadcrumbs, place some small pieces of butter on top, and bake for another half hour until the marrow is quite soft and a nice rich brown. Serve with brown gravy.

40. Purée of Walnuts.

Make a white sauce with 1-oz. butter, 1-oz. flour, ½-teacup of milk, add ½-pint of ground walnuts, ½-pint breadcrumbs, and 2 dessertspoons of milk, and beat well. About three-quarters-of-an-hour before serving, add the white of 1 egg stirred in lightly and pour into a mould. Steam for half-an-hour, serve with mashed potatoes.

41. Nut Croquettes.

Take ½-pint of mixed and shelled nuts, 4 or 5 mashed potatoes, 1 chopped and fried onion, and a pinch of mace. Chop the nuts, or pass through a nut-mill, and add them to the potato, with the onion and seasoning. Form into croquettes, brush over with egg, and cover with fine breadcrumbs and fry in boiling oil. Serve with bread sauce.

42. Mock Chicken Cutlets.

A tasty dish to be served with bread sauce is prepared as follows:—Run through the nut mill 2 cups of breadcrumbs and 1 good cup of shelled walnuts. Mix these together with a small piece of butter, a tablespoonful of grated onion juice, and a teaspoonful of mace. Melt a large teaspoonful of butter in a saucepan, with half a teaspoonful of flour and add gradually 2 cups of fresh milk; when this boils add the other ingredients, salt and pepper to taste, add a beaten egg, and when removed from the fire, a teaspoonful of lemon juice. Stir well and turn out into a dish to cool, then shape into cutlets, dip in egg, then in breadcrumbs, as usual, and fry crisp.

43. Mock Sweetbread Quenelles.

Put 1 pint of milk in a saucepan to boil with 1 onion chopped fine, when it boils add 3-ozs. of semolina stirring all the time, boil for 15 minutes, then add 1-oz. of breadcrumbs, 1-oz of butter, 1 egg, pepper and salt to taste. Mix well and steam in a buttered basin for half-an-hour, then cut out in pieces the shape of an egg (with a deep spoon), pile them in the centre of the dish, and pour thick white sauce over them, garnish with green peas, and carrots very finely chopped.

44. White Haricot Cutlets.

Skin and stew till quite tender ½-pint of white haricot beans in sufficient water to cover them. Add 2 small onions grated, 1 tablespoon of milk or cream, pepper and salt to taste. Simmer a little longer, and beat till quite smooth. Take off the fire, and add enough breadcrumbs to make fairly firm, form into cutlets, dip in egg, then in crumbs, and fry crisp. Serve with brown or tomato sauce.

45. Lentil Cutlets.

Take a teacup of Egyptian lentils; boil them in water sufficient to cover until tender. Add 3 grated onions, some chopped parsley and thyme, and enough breadcrumbs to make a stiff mixture. Turn on to large plates and flatten with a knife. Then cut into eight triangular sections and shape them like small cutlets. When cold, roll in egg, then in breadcrumbs, and fry crisp after inserting small pieces of macaroni into each pointed end. Serve with mint or tomato sauce, and with vegetables.

46. Mushroom Pie, with Gravy.

Take ¼-lb. butter beans, ¼-lb. mushrooms, 1-lb. chestnuts, 2 onions, 1 hard boiled egg, 1 teacupful tapioca (soaked overnight), some short crust pastry.

Fill a pie dish with alternate layers of above ingredients, with seasoning to taste; the onions and mushrooms should be fried, the chestnuts boiled and peeled, the butter beans cooked the day before until quite soft, and the egg cut into slices. Cover with the pastry made as follows:—½-lb. of flour, ¼-lb. nut butter, mixed with cold water. Brush over with beaten egg and bake.

GRAVY. Melt 1-oz. of butter in a saucepan, stir in a tablespoon of flour, and cook till a rich dark brown, stirring all the time, add half-a-pint of vegetable stock and being to the boil. Before serving add half-a-teaspoonful of Marmite.

47. Baked Nuttoria.

Open a tin of Nuttoria, cut into slices ½-inch in thickness, bake for an hour, well dressed with butter. Serve with vegetables and with rich gravy made from brown haricot beans, thickened with arrowroot, and flavoured with fried onion and a good piquant sauce (such as Brand's A1). Yorkshire pudding makes a suitable addition.

48. Lentil Croquettes.

Wash, pick and cook ¼-lb. lentils, with 1 or 2 onions to flavour. When cooked, add about 5-ozs. wholemeal breadcrumbs, a teaspoonful parsley, nutmeg, mace, salt and pepper, and 1 egg beaten. Mix well, and when cold form into balls. Dip in egg, then crumbs, and fry a golden brown. Serve with onion sauce and gravy.

49. Protose Cutlets.

Pound a tin of Protose with 1-oz. of fresh butter, some grated onion juice, parsley, thyme, salt and pepper, a few breadcrumbs, and a few drops of lemon juice. Roll the mixture on a floured board until about ½-inch thick, shape into cutlets, roll in egg, then in crumbs and fry. As Protose does not require previous cooking this is a very quickly prepared dish, and if a few tins are kept in stock it is always handy for emergencies. The cutlets may be fried without egg and breadcrumbs, simply rolled in a little flour, if one is very pressed for time. Serve with tomato or onion sauce, or a rich gravy.

50. Savoury Nut-Meat Steaks.

Cut some slices of Protose about 3/8-inch thick, and bake in a tin, basted with butter, for an hour. Roll in egg, then in crumbs, and fry in butter for a few minutes. Serve with fried forcemeat balls, red currant jelly, and brown haricot gravy flavoured with fried onion, cloves and some piquant sauce, thickened with arrowroot. Masked potatoes (placed round) complete this dish.

51. Nut-Meat à la Mode.

Take a tin of Nuttoria (½-lb.) and pass it through the nut-mill. Beat the whites and yolks of 4 eggs separately. Mix these with the nut-meat, adding 2-ozs. stale brown breadcrumbs, some grated onion, chopped parsley and herbs. Press into a basin and steam until well cooked. Serve with white parsley sauce thickened with arrowroot. This dish tastes exactly as if it were made with minced beef.

52. Nut-Meat Rissoles.

Put some Protose, Fibrose (brown), Nuttoria, or other nut-meat through the nut-mill before cooking. Fry slowly with some chopped onion. Cover with brown stock, and cook slowly until nearly all the gravy is absorbed. Then add breadcrumbs, herbs, seasoning, and a little butter, stir thoroughly over the fire, and set aside on a plate to cool. Form the mixture into small rolls, dip in egg, roll in breadcrumbs, and fry. Garnish with parsley, and serve with onion sauce or brown gravy.

53. Jugged Nuttose.

Bake some Nuttose (dressed with butter) for half-an-hour, in slices half-an-inch thick; then dip in egg and breadcrumbs, and fry. Also make some forcemeat balls by rubbing ½-oz. of butter in 5-ozs. of breadcrumbs, adding chopped lemon thyme, lemon peel and parsley, some pepper and salt, and 1 egg to bind; fry very brown. Cut up the Nuttose in quarter pieces and stew slowly in remainder of the bean stock with about 10 cloves. Garnish with sprays of parsley and the forcemeat balls. Serve with red currant jelly and mashed potatoes.

54. Nuttose Ragout.

A good way to prepare Nuttose is as follows:—Fry a teaspoonful of butter until quite brown, add flour until it absorbs the butter, add gradually any vegetable stock until a nice rich gravy results. Bring to the boil and add very thin slices of Nuttose. Stew very slowly for 1 hour, adding some Worcester or other sauce to taste. Garnish with mashed potatoes and serve with a green vegetable.

55. Minced Nut-meat.

Prepare a tin of Protose or other nut-meat by running it through a mincing machine, or mashing it with a fork, and stewing it in vegetable gravy. Serve with a border of green peas or beans, and with mashed potatoes placed round the outside of the dish. It is also nice served as follows, viz.:—Prepare as for minced meat. Boil a cupful of rice as for curry. When cooked stir in one teaspoonful of tomato sauce and seasoning. Put the mince in the centre of the dish with a wall of the rice and tomato round it.

56. Lentil and Potato Sausages.

Boil 5-ozs. lentils in very little water, so that when cooked all water is absorbed, then add 1 chopped and fried onion, a tiny pinch of herbs, pepper and salt, 4 boiled and mashed potatoes, and the *yolk* of 1 egg. Allow to cool a little, then flour the hands, and form into sausage shape. Brush over with white of egg and fry in boiling oil. Decorate with parsley and serve with a border of green peas.

57. Stuffed Yorkshire Pudding.

For the stuffing:—¼-lb. cooked lentils, 1 onion chopped and fried, a pinch of herbs, 2 tablespoonfuls of breadcrumbs, and seasoning.

For the batter:—¼-lb. of flour, ½-pint of milk, 1 egg.

Mix the batter and partly bake for 20 minutes; remove from oven, spread with stuffing, roll up carefully, return to oven and bake brown. Serve with apple sauce and brown gravy.

58. Mushroom and Potato Croquettes.

Take some stiff mashed potatoes. Make a stuffing with ¼-lb. minced and fried mushrooms, 2-ozs. chopped and cooked macaroni, and 1 tablespoonful breadcrumbs, moisten with a little beaten egg. Shape 2 rounds of potato, make a hollow in one, fill with the stuffing and press the other over it. Roll in egg, then in breadcrumbs, and fry crisp.

59. Mock Steak Pudding.

Take 1-lb. chestnuts, ¼-lb. mushrooms, 1 onion, 1-oz. butter, ½-pint stock, a few forcemeat balls, and 4-ozs. of pine kernels. Make a thick brown gravy with the butter, onion and stock, boil the chestnuts, remove the skins and husks and add them to the gravy, with pepper and salt to taste, simmer for 15 minutes. Line a buttered basin with a good crust (allowing 4-ozs. rolled and chopped pine kernels and ½-oz. butter to 8-ozs. flour) and put in a layer of the chestnut mixture, then a layer of chopped mushroom and forcemeat balls till the basin is quite full; cover with a thick crust and boil for 2½ hours.

60. Mock Chicken Rolls.

Take 1 cup brazil nuts, 2 cups breadcrumbs, 1 gill milk, 1 oz. butter, a little pepper and salt, mace, a few drops of lemon juice. Melt the butter and add the milk and flour to it, cook for a few minutes, add the breadcrumbs and ground nuts, then the other ingredients, mix well and turn over on a plate to cool. Form into rolls, dip into egg, then in breadcrumbs, and fry in boiling oil.

Serve with bread sauce and mashed potatoes.

61. Savoury Sausages.

Make of the same ingredients as in recipe No. 64. Pound well in a basin, season rather highly, add a few chopped mushrooms, and a little butter. Leave to get quite cold. Then form into sausages, with well-floured hands, brush over with beaten egg, and fry or bake till crisp and brown. They may need a little basting if they are baked.

62. Savoury Chestnut Mould.

Peel two dozen chestnuts and stew gently in vegetable stock until nearly soft. Now remove half the chestnuts, and continue to cook the remainder until quite soft, gradually reducing the stock. Mash the contents of the pan with a fork, then stir in 2 tablespoonfuls of breadcrumbs, 2-ozs. of butter, pepper and salt, 1 egg, and lastly the partly cooked chestnuts, cut into neat pieces. Well grease a basin or mould, pour in the mixture and steam three-quarters of an hour, and serve with brown gravy or onion sauce. The main point about this dish is to retain the flavour of the chestnut without the addition of herbs, &c., &c.

63. Walnut Pie.

(A Tasty Dish).

Put 4-ozs. of shelled walnuts through a mincer. Put a layer of boiled rice at the bottom of a buttered baking dish. Spread half the minced nuts evenly on top of the rice, then a layer of tomatoes, seasoned with onion, pepper and salt, mace, and ketchup, then another layer of rice, more nuts, etc., till the dish is nearly full. Cover thickly with breadcrumbs, pour melted butter over, and bake a nice brown. Serve with tomato sauce.

64. Savoury Lentil Roll.

Take 2 teacupfuls of boiled German lentils, put in a basin, and add a cupful of fine breadcrumbs, and about half as much mashed potatoes. Add any seasoning—ketchup, Worcester sauce—and a spoonful of melted butter. Mix well with a fork and bind with 1 or 2 beaten eggs, reserving a little for brushing over. Shape into a brick or oval, and press together as firmly as possible. Brush over with the remainder of the egg, put into a buttered tin and bake for half an hour. Serve with a garnish of beetroot or tomatoes.

65. Pine Kernel Timbale.

Well grease a basin and line it with partly cooked macaroni; start at the bottom of the basin, and coil each piece carefully round, all touching, until the basin is completely lined. Now carefully fill with the following farce:— Fry in 2-ozs. of butter two or three chopped onions, then add about 6-ozs. of pine-kernels, having first ground them in a nut-mill, continue frying till a pale brown, then turn into a basin and add about ½-lb. breadcrumbs, pepper and salt, and 2 eggs. Cover the basin with greased paper and steam one hour. Remove carefully from the basin and pour round a nice brown gravy.

SIMPLE SAVOURY DISHES.

66. Macaroni Napolitaine.

Boil ½-lb. best quality macaroni (large) in plenty of water, strain and place on a dish; take a dessertspoonful of cornflour, mix thoroughly with a little milk, add milk to make half a pint, boil until it thickens, add half an ounce of grated cheese, a small knob of butter, and a few tablespoonfuls of tomato sauce or tomato conserve. The tomato sauce can be made by slicing 4 tomatoes and cooking them in a saucepan with a little batter and chopped onion. Pass through a strainer. Pour the sauce over the macaroni or serve in a sauce boat.

67. Macaroni à la Turque.

Boil ¼-lb. of macaroni until *slightly* tender, and add ½-lb. of grated breadcrumbs, 1 large onion (grated), 2 large tablespoons of parsley, some grated nutmeg, ½-pint milk, and 1 egg (beaten). Chop the macaroni and mix all well together and steam in a basin or in moulds for 1 or 1½ hours. Serve with thin white sauce or brown gravy (poured over the mould).

68. Macaroni Cutlets.

Boil ¼-lb. macaroni (Spaghetti) in water, not making it too tender; chop slightly, add 6-ozs. breadcrumbs, some chopped fried onions, a teaspoonful of lemon thyme, and parsley, a couple of tomatoes (fried in saucepan after onions), and 1 egg to bind. Mix, roll in flour, shape into cutlets, fry until crisp and brown. Serve with piquant or tomato sauce.

69. Savoury Macaroni.

Boil some macaroni for half an hour, drain well and add 1-oz. butter, 1 beaten egg, pepper and salt, 1 peeled and sliced tomato. Heat all thoroughly together and serve.

70. Creamed Macaroni.

Break ¼-lb. macaroni into 1-inch pieces, drop them into 2-qts. of *boiling* water, (salted), boil till tender. Drain and place in a dish. At serving time put into a pan a tablespoon of butter, when melted, a tablespoon of flour, rub until well mixed, then add ½-pint of milk, stir until it bubbles; a little cayenne to be added, then put in the macaroni and heat thoroughly, and just at the last, stir in ¼-lb. of grated cheese (not quite half ought to be Parmesan and the rest a good fresh cheese).

71. Macaroni and Tomato Pudding.

Boil some macaroni and mix with it 3-ozs. of grated cheese, 4 peeled and sliced tomatoes, a little chopped parsley, and half a teacup of milk. Place in a pie-dish and cover with a thick layer of fine breadcrumbs and a few knobs of butter; season to taste. Bake until nicely browned. The addition of a grated onion is considered an improvement by many persons.

72. How to Cook Rice.

First boil the water, then put the rice in, and keep it on the boil for twelve minutes; if it wants to boil over just lift the lid of saucepan to let the steam escape. After boiling strain in a strainer, and steam it when wanted for use.

To steam the boiled rice, put it in a colander and stand the colander in a saucepan containing a little boiling water, so that the colander and rice are clear of the water, put saucepan on the hot plate, and the steam from the water will dry and separate out each grain of rice and make it flakey.

Savoury rice dishes can be made more rich in proteid, and more tasty, by adding a few teaspoons of Emprote.

73. Rice (Milanese).

(Specially recommended).

Boil 6-ozs. of unpolished rice in a double saucepan until tender. Fry a chopped onion brown, then add 2 peeled tomatoes and cook until soft, add this to the rice with the yolks of 2 eggs, ½-teaspoonful of salt, and 1½-ozs. of Parmesan or grated cheese. Mix well together and serve with brown gravy. This makes a most tasty and nutritious dish.

74. Rice alla Romana.

Boil 6-ozs. of unpolished rice with a clove of garlic. Fry 4 peeled tomatoes in 1-oz. butter. Add this to the rice with the yolk of 1 egg, ½-teaspoonful of salt, and 1-oz. of Parmesan or grated cheese. Stir and serve with tomato sauce, or garnish with baked tomatoes. This dish is equally suitable for lunch, dinner, or supper; it is a 'complete' type of food, and it is much appreciated. The flavour can easily be varied.

75. Savoury Rice.

Boil ¼-lb. of rice till quite soft, add a teaspoonful of chopped parsley, a little grated lemon rind, 4-ozs. grated cheese, 1 tablespoonful of milk and a little butter, mix well and put into scollop shells, sprinkle over with breadcrumbs and bake for 20 minutes.

76. proteid Rice Cutlets.

Delicious rice cutlets can be made as follows:—Fry 2 grated onions brown, then add 2 tomatoes in the same pan and cook till tender. Cook a large cupful of rice in a double saucepan, turn it into a basin, add the onions and tomatoes, a teaspoonful of chopped parsley, 2-ozs. of breadcrumbs, 2-ozs. of Emprote, and pepper and salt to taste. Mix well, turn out on plates and smooth with a wet knife, cut into fingers and fry crisp in egg and breadcrumbs. Serve with tomato sauce or brown gravy.

77. Sicilian Rice.

Fry in 1-oz. butter, one good handful of chopped parsley and one finely chopped onion, until the latter is a pale brown colour; now add equal quantities of boiled rice and nicely cooked cabbage or sprouts (chopped), pepper and salt, and a small teaspoonful of sugar. Mix all together and heat thoroughly. Serve.

78. Curried Rice and Peas.

(An Indian Dish).

Cook some rice in a jar until nicely swollen, put it in a saucepan, add one or two fried onions (and some young carrots chopped fine if desired), some vegetable stock, a dessertspoonful of Lazenby's Mango chutney, and 1 or 2 teaspoonfuls of Stembridge's curry paste, until the rice has a rich curry flavour, to taste. Warm ½-pint of small French green peas (use fresh ones in season) with sugar and mint, pour them in the centre of the dish, place the curried rice round them and garnish with small fingers of pastry. Serve with fried potatoes and cauliflower. This dish is easily made and very easy of digestion.

79. Risi Piselli.

(A Popular Italian Dish).

Fry some finely chopped parsley and onion till the latter is a light-brown colour. Have ready equal quantities of cooked rice and young green peas, boiled separately (let the rice be dry, well cooked, and each grain separate), add these to the onions and parsley, and stir well together in the pan. Serve very hot.

80. Rice and Tomato Rissoles.

Fry 2 onions brown, then add 4 peeled tomatoes, cook till tender, turn into a bowl and chop finely with some parsley and thyme. At the same time cook a small cupful of rice in a double pan. Mix this with the onions, etc., with pepper and salt, and 2-ozs. of breadcrumbs. Mix well, then put on plates, smooth over, and when quite cold cut into rissoles, egg, then crumb and fry. Serve with a rich brown gravy.

81. A Simple Omelette.

Take 2 eggs, 1 teaspoon chopped parsley, a little chopped onion, pepper and salt. Beat the yolks and whites separately and then add the other ingredients. Heat some butter in a frying pan until very hot, then pour in the mixture and keep putting a knife round the outside to prevent the omelette adhering, and to make the uncooked centre flow towards the rim. When nicely set fold and serve on a hot plate.

82. Omelette aux Tomates.

Take 3 eggs, ¼-pt. of milk, a teaspoonful chopped parsley, and a taste of grated onion juice, pepper and salt. Whisk all in a basin so as to mix thoroughly. Heat 1-oz. of butter in a frying-pan, then pour in the mixture and keep putting the knife round the outside to prevent the omelette adhering, and to make the uncooked centre flow towards the rim. When nicely set, fold and serve on a hot dish, either with tomato sauce, or garnished with baked tomatoes.

83. Eggs Florentine.

Boil some spinach in water containing a pinch of salt and soda, for about 10 minutes. Strain well, rub through a sieve, and add a well-beaten egg. Arrange in a fireproof dish, a thin layer in the centre and a good ridge all round, and put into the oven for about 10 minutes. Now poach a few eggs and lay in the centre, and sprinkle some Parmesan cheese over all, add some cheese sauce.

84. Eggs à la Crême.

Place a large tablespoonful of cream in each of several small fireproof china baking or soufflé dishes (about 3½-inches in diameter). Break an egg in each one, and steam them in a frying pan in water 1 inch deep until well cooked. Some persons who cannot digest lightly cooked eggs can safely take them if quite hard.

85. Mayonnaise Eggs.

Boil the eggs hard, which takes about 15 minutes, then put them in cold water; when cold, shell them and cut a piece off the end of each so that they will stand upright on the dish; pour thick mayonnaise sauce over them and sprinkle with chopped capers.

86. Eggs à l'Italienne.

Boil ¼-lb. of spaghetti in water, adding some tomato purée or conserve, and spread it on a dish. Poach 4 eggs and lay them on the spaghetti, sprinkle finely chopped parsley over the eggs and decorate the dish with fried croûtons.

87. Omelette aux Fines Herbes.

Melt 1-oz. of butter in a perfectly dry frying pan. Beat the yolks of 3 eggs with some finely chopped parsley and a pinch of garlic powder, pepper and salt. When the butter boils pour in the egg and stir until it commences to set. Then pour in the whites of the eggs (previously beaten to a stiff froth). When cooked fold the omelette and turn on to a very hot dish. Cover at once and serve.

88. Scrambled Eggs and Tomatoes.

Peel 4 large tomatoes after dipping them in scalding water, slice and stew them in a little butter for a few minutes; beat 2 eggs, add them to the tomatoes, and scramble them until the egg is cooked. Serve on toast. Green peas may be used for this dish instead of tomatoes.

89. Oeufs Farcie en Aspic.

Boil 4 eggs hard and remove the shells and take out the yolks, beat them in a bowl, and then add 2 teaspoons of salad oil and a little chopped parsley and thyme, a few breadcrumbs, pepper and salt, mix all well and fill in each white half, even over with a knife, and glaze. Serve with Salad and Mayonnaise Sauce.

90. Spinach and Eggs.

Take 3 or 4-lbs. of spinach, boil it in plenty of water with a pinch of soda and salt for 10 minutes, press through a strainer, and then rub through a wire sieve; place it in a saucepan with a small piece of butter and a tablespoonful of milk, stir well whilst being warmed up, and serve on buttered toast or fried bread, garnish with fingers of pastry. Rub 2 hard boiled eggs through a sieve and spread on the top. Decorate with the white of the eggs when sliced.

91. Spinach à la Crême.

Prepare the spinach as described above, but instead of adding butter and milk, add 2 or 3 tablespoons of cream. Stir well and serve with fingers of fried bread or pastry. Omit the garnishing of eggs.

92. Spinach Soufflé.

Cook some spinach (see recipe 90), pass it through sieve and add 2 or 3 well beaten eggs and a small amount of milk, with pepper and salt. Mix it thoroughly, put it in well buttered soufflé dishes and bake for 10 minutes. This makes a simple yet tasty entrée.

93. Green Pea Soufflé.

Pass some cooked green peas through a sieve, add pepper and salt, a teaspoonful of sugar, a very little milk, and the yolks of 2 or 3 eggs, according to quantity of peas. Beat the whites of eggs till a stiff froth, add to the mixture and bake quickly in an oiled soufflé dish or small cases.

94. Chestnut Soufflé.

Boil 1-lb of chestnuts until they are quite soft, remove the skins and pass through a nut-mill, moisten with ¼-pt. of milk and ½-oz. butter (melted), add pepper and salt, the yolks of 3 eggs and lastly the whites, beaten to a stiff froth. Pour into a greased soufflé dish and bake quickly.

95. Lentil Soufflé.

Cook 2-ozs. of lentils in very little water (so that when cooked the moisture is absorbed), add 1-oz. of butter, pepper and salt, 1 tablespoonful of milk, and the yolks of 3 eggs. Beat the whites to a stiff froth and fold lightly into the mixture. Pour into an oiled soufflé dish and bake quickly.

96. Asparagus Soufflé.

Take some asparagus (previously boiled) and rub it through a sieve. Add 2 or 3 well beaten eggs and a small quantity of milk, with pepper and salt. Beat it well and put in buttered soufflé dishes and bake for 10 minutes. This makes a tasty course for a luncheon or dinner, and also a simple supper dish.

97. Cabbage Soufflé.

Take some well-cooked cabbage or Brussels sprouts, pass through a sieve, add pepper and salt, a little milk, and well beat in the yolks of 2 or 3 eggs. Beat the whites to a stiff froth and stir lightly into the mixture. Pour into the soufflé dish in which has been melted a small piece of butter. Bake quickly in a good oven.

98. Savoury Rissoles.

Equal quantities of mashed wholemeal bread and boiled rice, add a little boiled onion minced fine, some pepper, salt and butter. Mix, roll into shape, or pass through a sausage machine, dredge with flour, dip in batter, and fry crisp. A great variety can be made by introducing lentils, macaroni or haricots, with herbs, fried onions, breadcrumbs, etc., and an egg.

99. Kedgeree.

Two cups of boiled rice, 2 hard boiled eggs, 1-oz. butter, 1 onion, 1-oz. sultanas, pepper and salt. Fry the onion in the butter till brown, then add the rice, eggs, and seasoning, mix well and serve very hot.

100. Savoury Cheese Rissoles.

Put ½-pint of hot water and 2-ozs. butter in a saucepan and bring to the boil, sift in slowly 5-ozs. of flour and cook this mixture thoroughly until it will leave the pan clean. Take it off the fire and add a little cayenne, finely chopped parsley, 4-ozs. breadcrumbs, 2-ozs. grated cheese, and 1 egg beaten in separately. When the mixture is quite cool, roll it into balls with flour and fry them. Decorate the dish with parsley and serve hot with a garnish of mashed potatoes. A brown sauce is an improvement.

101. A Corsican Dish.

Take 1-lb. Brussels sprouts, and sauté them, 1-lb. chestnuts, boil and peel them, and then fry in butter. Pile in centre of dish and surround with the sprouts. Decorate with croûtons and serve hot.

102. Brussels Sprouts Sauté.

Blanch the sprouts and drain well. Put into a wide saucepan with some butter and seasoning. Place on a hot fire and shake frequently for five minutes. Serve hot.

103. Spinach Fritters.

Chop finely, or pass through a sieve, 1-lb. of cooked spinach, season with salt and pepper and add the yolk of 1 egg and sufficient breadcrumbs to make the mixture stiff. Form into flat, round cakes, dip into frying batter and cook in boiling fat. Serve with a garnish of scrambled eggs.

104. Baked Stuffed Tomatoes.

Remove the centre from half a dozen tomatoes, mince this and add some chopped parsley, ¼-lb. grated nuts, 2-ozs. breadcrumbs, pepper and salt to taste and one egg. Fill the tomatoes with this mixture and bake for half an hour, first placing a small piece of butter on each tomato.

105. A Breakfast Dish.

Take some large tomatoes, cut them in halves and scoop out the inside. Break some eggs and put each in a cup, and slide one egg into each half tomato. Put a little chopped parsley on each, and bake in the oven until the white of the egg is set. Serve on rounds of toast.

106. Vegetable Marrow Stuffed.

Grate some nuts, add the same quantity of breadcrumbs, season, bind with one egg. Take a small marrow, cut in halves, scoop out the seeds, put in the stuffing, place it in a cloth upright in a saucepan with water, and steam for one hour.

107. Tomatoes au Gratin.

Take some large tomatoes, cut in halves, take out the pulp. Make a stuffing of nut-meat, or of grated nuts, bind with one egg, and fill up the tomatoes. Sprinkle a little grated cheese and breadcrumbs and a dab of butter on each tomato round. Place in a tin, and bake in the oven for twenty minutes, and serve on croûtons.

108. Brussels Sprouts à la Simone.

(An Italian dish)

Wash and boil the sprouts in the usual way, drain dry, and put them in a hot dish. Have ready a sauce made with 2-ozs. of butter, 2 tablespoonfuls of flour, add ½ a pint of stock and stir till it boils; just before serving add a good sprinkling of pepper and the juice of half a lemon; pour the sauce over the sprouts and serve.

109. Potato Purée.

Boil some large potatoes until soft, strain off the water, and dry them, mash with a silver fork, mix in a little salt and pepper, some butter and a cupful of hot milk, beat well until the mixture is quite smooth and creamy. Serve very hot.

110. Onions à la Mode Francaise.

Take some Spanish onions, peel them, and make a hole in the centre, and put in each onion a small piece of butter and one lump of sugar. Add a little pepper and salt, and simmer in a covered stewpan for 2 hours. The onions should then be cooked, and surrounded with a rich gravy of their own.

111. Escalloped Potatoes.

Mix a pint and a half of cold potatoes cut in cubes and seasoned with salt, and a pint of cream sauce. Put the mixture in shallow baking dish, cover with grated breadcrumbs, and dot with butter. Bake half an hour in moderate oven.

112. Baked Vegetable Marrow.

Mix together ½-oz. of butter with 5-ozs. breadcrumbs, rubbing it well in. Add a fried onion, some parsley and thyme, some sage and some lemon rind, and bind with an egg. Scoop out the marrow, and place the stuffing in quite dry; then steam in a cloth. Dress with brown gravy and fried breadcrumbs, and place for a few minutes in a hot oven.

113. Milanese Croquettes.

Pass 2 hard boiled eggs through a sieve, then mix with 3 or 4-ozs. of cold mashed potatoes. Add pepper and salt to taste, and nutmeg. Form into little rolls and dip into egg and breadcrumbs, then fry crisp.

114. Green Lentil Cutlets.

Slice and fry till brown 1 large onion, then add ½-pint of green lentils (well washed), and cover with water or stock, bring to the boil, and simmer gently till quite tender. Rub through a sieve to keep back the skins; add 2-ozs. of breadcrumbs, 1-oz. mashed potatoes, a little chopped parsley and some mushroom ketchup, salt and pepper to taste. Make into cutlet shapes, roll in flour, or egg and breadcrumbs, and fry crisp. Serve with brown gravy.

115. Chestnut and Mushroom Pudding.

Line a pudding basin with good short pastry, then fill it with layers of white haricots (skinned and steamed till nearly tender), fried onion, tapioca, (previously soaked for 1 or 2 hours in cold water), finely chopped parsley, fried mushrooms, and some chestnuts (skinned and boiled till nearly tender), also a sprinkling of salt and pepper between the layers. Pour over all some nicely seasoned mushroom gravy; cover with pastry, tie a floured cloth over it, and steam for 3 hours.

116. Savoury Golden Marbles.

Take nearly ½-pt. of white haricot beans, cooked and pulped through a sieve, and add 2-ozs. of breadcrumbs, 2-ozs. of mashed potatoes, a small onion finely minced, and pepper and salt to taste. Add 1 beaten egg. Mix thoroughly, and form into marbles. Coat with the remainder of the egg, toss in fine breadcrumbs, and fry crisp and light brown.

117. Potato Croquettes.

Boil 2-lbs. of potatoes, well dry them, mash thoroughly with ½-oz. butter and 1 beaten egg. Lay on a dish until cold. Shape into balls, dip in egg and breadcrumbs, and fry crisp.

118. Curried Lentils.

Stew some green lentils in vegetable stock, and when quite soft stir in a teaspoonful of Stembridge's curry paste, a fried onion, a chopped apple, and some chutney. Mix it well. Serve with a border of boiled rice, and fingers of pastry or fried bread, and some chipped potatoes.

119. Yorkshire Savoury Pudding.

Take 3 eggs, 5 tablespoons of flour, 1 pint of milk, 1 large onion, pepper and salt to taste. Beat the whites of the eggs to a stiff froth, mix the yolks with the milk, flour and condiments, lightly mix in the whites and pour into one or two well greased pudding tins which should have been made hot. Bake 20 minutes. The pudding should not be more than three-eighths of an inch in thickness, and should be of a nice brown colour.

120. Cauliflower (au Gratin).

Boil 1 or 2 cauliflowers (after removing leaves) until tender. Strain off the water and place on a dish. Cover with grated cheese, some white sauce and some fried breadcrumbs. Add some knobs of butter and bake until a nice brown. This dish is very savoury, and is useful for supper or as a separate course for dinner.

121. Curried Cauliflower.

Wash a nice fresh cauliflower carefully, then boil it in salted water until it is quite tender, be careful that it does not break, drain it well from the water, place it in a hot dish, arrange it in a neat compact shape, pressing it gently together with a nice clean cloth, pour over some curry sauce and serve with or without a rice border.

122. Grilled Tomatoes.

Halve some ripe tomatoes, place them in a frying pan with a teacupful of water, put a small piece of butter on each piece. Cook them until tender. Serve on toast. Poached eggs or mushrooms are a nice addition to this dish.

123. Neapolitan Sausages.

Soak 2 tablespoons of tapioca for 1 hour or more, then add ½-lb. of breadcrumbs, 1 hard boiled egg, 2 tablespoons of olive oil, 1 teaspoonful chopped parsley, and a little thyme, and pepper and salt to taste. Mix well with half a raw egg. Make into sausage shape, roll in egg, then in breadcrumbs, and fry crisp, or bake in a tin with a little butter in a sharp oven. Serve with brown gravy and apple sauce.

124. Lentil Pudding.

Stew some green lentils until soft; stir in some of Stembridge's curry paste and add chutney to taste. Season with salt and butter, cover with mashed potatoes and bake.

125. Savoury Rice Pudding.

Put 1 teacupful of rice in a medium sized pie dish, and fill it with milk; chop finely or grate 4 small onions, beat 1 egg, mix altogether, add a tablespoonful of chopped parsley and a little salt; bake in a slow oven. After 20 minutes, stir the pudding thoroughly, adding a small piece of butter, and a little more milk if necessary.

126. Croûtes a la Valencia.

Two ozs. almonds, 1 hard boiled egg, 1 oz. fresh butter, 1 teaspoonful olive oil, salt and pepper, 8 small rounds of fried bread. Blanch the almonds and fry them slowly in the oil till a golden brown, place on kitchen paper and sprinkle with salt. Allow these to get cold. Drain the rest of the nuts, and pound them in a mortar till quite fine, add the egg and butter, and season well. Pound all together till quite smooth, then pile up on the rounds of bread, and arrange 3 of the salted almonds on each.

127. Frittamix Rissoles.

Take ½-lb. of frittamix (Mapleton's), 2-ozs. of fine stale breadcrumbs and 1-oz. of butter. Mix all together with some boiling water and make into rissoles or sausages, egg and breadcrumb them and fry crisp in boiling Nutter.

128. Marmite Toast.

(A good breakfast dish).

Spread some Marmite on rounds of white bread, fry till they are crisp, and serve with scrambled eggs piled on each round, or piled in a dish with fried eggs.

129. Salted Almonds.

Heat a dessertspoonful of butter in a frying pan till it smokes, place some blanched almonds in it, sprinkle lightly with salt and pepper, or red pepper if liked, shake the pan till the almonds are *slightly* brown, place on paper to drain, and serve.

130. Chestnut Stew.

Take 1-lb. chestnuts, 1½-ozs. oil or butter, 1 tablespoonful flour, 1 pt. milk, 1 yolk of egg, 1 tablespoonful of chopped parsley. Add pepper and salt. Boil the chestnuts for ¼-hour, then place in hot oven for 5 minutes, when the skins will be easy to remove. Put the oil into a saucepan and in it fry the chestnuts for a few minutes, stir in 1 tablespoonful of flour, add the milk gradually with pepper and salt, and let the whole simmer gently for half an hour. Just before serving, add the parsley chopped fine. The yolk of an egg may also be added to give greater richness, but in this case do not let it boil again. This dish is both nutritious and tasty.

COLD LUNCHEON DISHES

(For Hot Luncheon Dishes see previous section of Recipes).

131. Oeufs Farcie en Aspic.

Boil 4 eggs hard and remove the shells, and take out the yolks; beat them in a bowl, and then add 2 teaspoons of salad oil and a little chopped parsley and thyme, a few breadcrumbs, pepper and salt. Mix all well and fill in each white half, even over with a knife, and glaze. Serve with Salad and Mayonnaise sauce.

132. Nut Galantine.

Take ½-lb. ground walnuts, ¼-lb. cooked spaghetti, 2 onions, 1 small tomato, 1-oz. butter, 1 dessertspoonful of Carnos, a little stock, pepper and salt to taste. Fry the onions and tomato in the butter, and then add the other ingredients and simmer for 15 minutes. Put into a greased mould, cover with a greased paper, and bake in a slow oven for 1 hour. Turn out when cold and serve with salad and Mayonnaise sauce. This dish may be served hot as a roast with red currant jelly and browned potatoes.

133. Galantine alla Bolognese.

Steam ½-pint of rice, fry 12 mushrooms and 6 small onions, add ½-pint breadcrumbs, and put all through the sausage mill; add 2 well beaten eggs, pepper and salt, and a pinch of mixed spice. Put the mixture in buttered paper and shape it like a bolster, fastening the ends with white of egg. Tie it in a cloth and steam for 1½ hours, then take it off the fire and leave it to cool. Before serving take off the paper, then glaze with aspic. Decorate with chopped hard-boiled eggs, or beetroot and carrot cut in shapes; and serve with chutney or salad sauce.

134. Aspic Jelly.

Take 2 pints of cold water, ¼-oz. agar-agar (vegetable gelatine), 1 lemon, some pepper and salt, a pinch of cayenne, and 2 tablespoons of Tarragon vinegar. Soak the agar 2 hours in 1-pt. of the water, then add the other ingredients, with some Worcester sauce to darken it, add the white of an egg and the shell, put over a slow fire till the agar is dissolved, then boil 2 or 3 minutes, and strain through a coarse flannel.

135. Mock Lobster Shapes.

Put the yolks of 4 hard-boiled eggs through a sieve, add by degrees 4 tablespoonfuls of salad oil. When a perfectly smooth paste is formed; add 1 teaspoonful of Tarragon vinegar, 1 teaspoonful of malt vinegar, 1 gill of cool jelly, 1 gill cream. Have ready about 3-ozs. boiled haricot beans, chop them coarsely and add to the mixture, put into small moulds. When set, turn out and glaze.

136. Raised Pie.

Line a pie-mould with good short crust, then fill with the following mixture: —Omelette made with 2 eggs, 2-ozs. chopped macaroni, a little grated onion, chopped parsley, pepper and salt; 5 or 6 tomatoes peeled and fried in a little butter, seasoned with a pinch of sugar, pepper and salt, and thickened with 2 eggs scrambled in them. Leave these till cold, fit into the pie; cover, brush with egg, and bake in a good hot oven at first, then slowly for about an hour. Garnish with parsley and serve cold or hot.

137. Green Pea Galantine.

Pass 1 pint of green peas (cooked) through a sieve, add 1 small grated onion, some chopped mint, ¼-lb. pine kernel nut-meat (first passing it through a mill), 2-ozs. tapioca, which has been soaked overnight in cold water, pepper and salt, and ¼-lb. breadcrumbs. Mix well and add 1 raw egg. Put into a greased mould or pie dish and bake in a slow oven ¾ of an hour. Turn out when cold and serve with salad.

138. Picnic Brawn.

Fry 1 onion, 1 lump of sugar, in a little butter till quite brown, add 2 tablespoonfuls of Marmite, ¾-pint of water. Dissolve ½-oz. of gelatine in a little water and add to the gravy. Simmer all together for 15 minutes and strain, then add some cooked cold vegetables, a little cooked macaroni, and 1 hard-boiled egg chopped finely. Pepper and salt to taste, wet a mould with cold water and pour the mixture in to set. Turn out when cold and quite firm. Decorate with carrots, etc., cut into shape, and a white paper frill.

139. Tomato Galantine.

Six peeled tomatoes, 3 tablespoons of cooked macaroni, 3 onions chopped and fried, ½-cup tapioca (soaked in cold water), nearly a cup of bread which has been soaked in cold water, drained and fried in the pan after the onions; mix all with 1 unbeaten egg, pour into a greased mould which is decorated with hard-boiled egg, cover with greased paper and bake in a slow oven till set. Eat cold with salad.

140. Nut-Meat Galantine.

Take ½-lb. Protose, ¼-lb. spaghetti (cooked), 8 large chestnuts (boiled and peeled), and 2 onions fried; put these through a sausage machine and add ½-cupful of tapioca which has been soaked in cold water, 1-oz. of butter broken into small pieces, and pepper and salt to taste. Mix well, then put into a greased mould. Cover with greased paper, and bake in a slow oven 1 hour. Turn out when cold and serve with salad and mayonnaise.

141. Tomato Mayonnaise.

Peel and slice 6 good tomatoes, place them in a dish and cover them with Mayonnaise sauce; let them stand for a few hours. Serve after sprinkling some finely chopped parsley over the top. This dish tastes nice with Protose rolls, or cheese, &c.

142. Nut-Meat Rolls.

Prepare pastry as usual for sausage rolls, either short or puffy. The filling mixture is made just as for the Nut-Meat Rissoles (52), with the addition of a few breadcrumbs. Roll the mixture between the fingers into the shape of a sausage, and proceed just as usual. Brush with egg and bake in a quick oven.

143. Protose Luncheon Rolls.

Break up with a fork ½-lb. of Protose, add to this some chopped parsley, 2 peeled tomatoes, crumbs, pepper and salt, and a few drops of A1 sauce. Mix thoroughly. Have ready some short pastry, cut into squares, place a little of the mixture in each, fold in the usual way. Brush over with egg and bake in a quick oven.

144. Potted White Haricots.

(A Substitute for Potted Chicken.)

Stew a cupful of white haricots with 6 onions and water to cover them, until perfectly soft. Rub through a wire sieve or potato masher. Add 3-ozs. of mashed potato, 6-ozs. of brown breadcrumbs, 1-oz. of butter, 1-oz. grated cheese, and an eggspoonful of mustard. Mix well with pestle and mortar and fill small pots, cover with melted butter.

145. Potted Lentil Savoury.

Take ¼-lb. lentils (cooked), 3-ozs. mashed potato, 2-ozs. breadcrumbs, 1 egg (beaten), chopped parsley, a little onion juice, salt and pepper, and 1-oz. butter. Put all in a pan and mix well together, with 2-ozs. of grated cheese, stirring all the time. When cooked, turn into a mortar, pound well and press into potting dishes and melt butter over the top. This makes excellent sandwiches with a little mustard spread on it.

146. Nut Sandwiches.

Flake some Brazil or other nuts and spread a thin layer in some bread and butter sandwiches which have been dressed with honey or jam. Almonds can be used if preferred, and curry powder instead of preserve, if they are preferred savoury instead of sweet.

147. Tomato or Egg Sandwiches.

Make sandwiches by spreading tomato paste between slices of bread and butter. A dish of mustard and cress sandwiches should be served with them. Sieved hard-boiled eggs, with a pinch of herbs, make good sandwiches also.

148. Egg and Cress Sandwiches.

Take some eggs, boiled hard; chop very fine and place between some rounds of white bread, spread a little Mayonnaise sauce on them and a layer of chopped cress. The rounds of bread should be cut out with a cutter. Pile the sandwiches on a dish and decorate with parsley, and a little chopped yolk of the eggs.

149. Cabbage Salad.

Two eggs well beaten, 6 tablespoonfuls of cream, ½-teaspoon of salt, 6 teaspoons of vinegar, and a small piece of butter. Put on the fire and cook, stirring continually until quite thick. Prepare a half head of cabbage chopped fine, sprinkled with salt. Add to the dressing when cold 2 tablespoonfuls of cream, and pour over the cabbage.

150. Potted Haricot Savoury.

Put a good breakfastcupful of brown beans, with a few onions, into a brown stew-jar, and cover with a quart, or rather more, of water. Place in a slow oven and cook until the beans crack, and the liquid will then have become a rich brown colour. After the liquid has been poured from the beans (to be used as stock or for haricot tea) rub them through a sieve or masher. To 7-ozs. of the pulp, add 3-ozs. mashed potato, 3-ozs. brown breadcrumbs, and 1½-ozs. butter; salt, pepper, nutmeg and mace to taste, and a little fried onion if liked. Put all in a pan and stir till hot, add 1 beaten egg, and cook until the mixture leaves the sides of the pan, but do not let it get too stiff. Press into potting dishes as usual.

151. Cheese and Tomato Paste.

Take ½-lb. Cheddar cheese, flake it, then take 2 good sized tomatoes, peel them by placing them in hot water for a few minutes. Put the tomatoes into a basin, chop and beat them into a pulp, add pepper and a little chopped parsley, mint, and thyme. Mix the tomato pulp with the grated cheese and beat well together until a paste is produced. Press into small soufflé dishes.

152. Potted Haricot Meat.

Stew some brown haricot beans for several hours (saving the liquor for stock). Pass them through a sieve, mix with them some brown breadcrumbs, a finely chopped raw onion, parsley, a little thyme and a ¼-oz. of butter; pepper and salt to taste. Heat all together in a saucepan for 10 minutes; pour into jars, and cover with melted butter. This is a useful dish for breakfast, supper, or when travelling.

153. Savoury Protose Pudding.

Make a good stuffing of 1-lb. wholemeal breadcrumbs, sweet herbs, ¼-lb. butter, chopped parsley, peel of 1 lemon, chopped fine, and pepper and salt to taste. Bind with 2 or 3 eggs. Thickly line a well-greased pie dish with the stuffing, then press into the middle a tin of Protose (minced or machined). Thickly cover over with stuffing. Put little pieces of butter or nucoline on top, cover with a tin and bake in slow oven an hour or an hour and a half. This makes a savoury dish, when cold, with a good salad.

154. Potted Tomato Paste.

Three tomatoes, 1 egg, 2-ozs. grated cheese, 4-ozs. breadcrumbs, ½-oz. butter, 1 small onion minced fine, pepper and celery salt. Peel the tomatoes and cut them up in a small saucepan with the butter and onion; when tender, mash smoothly and add the egg. Stir quickly until it becomes thick; add the cheese and breadcrumbs last, when off the fire. Turn into a pot and cover with butter.

155. Delicious Milk Cheese.

Make 1 gallon of rich milk just lukewarm, add the juice of 3 lemons, or 2 tablespoons of French Wine Vinegar, and stir well. Set aside till curd and whey are separated; now pour into a cheese cloth with a basin underneath to catch the whey. Let it hang (after tying up) until well drained, then place between two plates, or in a flat colander, with a weight on top, or in a cheese press, until firmly set.

156. A Good Salad Dressing.

Rub an eggspoonful of mustard, salt and sugar in a teaspoonful of olive oil and cream, until the mixture is quite smooth. Then rub the yolk of a hard-boiled egg in the paste, and keep it free from lumps. Pour in a dessertspoonful of vinegar, stirring slowly all the time. Add a teacupful of rich milk or some cream. Serve.

GRAVIES AND SAUCES.

A great variety of savoury and nutritious gravies can be made from vegetable stock, with the usual thickening, (arrowroot is best), a pinch of salt and pepper, seasoning, and a lump of butter. Brown haricot broth is the best stock (Recipe 5). The addition of Nutril, Wintox, Mapleton's Gravy Essence, or Marmite gives flavour and increases the nourishing quality.

It is very desirable that the gravy or sauce served with certain vegetarian dishes should be piquante in taste and of a nice flavour. It is worth while to take some trouble to achieve this result, because many dishes that are plain and perhaps somewhat tasteless in themselves are made quite savoury and enjoyable by the addition of a piquante dressing. Brand's A1 sauce is a good example of such piquancy, and is also useful in making sauces in the home, as a few teaspoons of it will often give an unique flavour to a simple gravy that is lacking in this respect.

157. Walnut Gravy.

Take about 4-ozs. of shelled walnuts, put them through the nut mill, and place in a small pan in which you have previously made hot 1-oz. of butter. Fry until the walnut is dark brown, *stirring well* all the time to prevent burning. Pour on a pint of stock, or water if no stock is at hand, and let it simmer slowly until just before serving. Then add 1-oz. of flour to thicken, some seasoning, and a few drops of onion or some tomato sauce. This makes a most rich and savoury gravy—especially if a little nut butter is added.

158. Curry Gravy.

In the cold weather, dishes which contain curry are seasonable and are generally appreciated. The following recipe for a curry gravy will prove useful to many readers, as it makes a capital addition to plain boiled rice or many other dishes. Fry 2 onions, minced in some butter until they are quite brown. Then sift in some flour and let it brown also. Add slowly some vegetable stock or water, two minced apples, a teaspoonful of curry paste (Stembridge's is good), a teaspoonful of vinegar, and a dessertspoonful each of tomato sauce and chutney. Stir and serve.

159. Gravy Piquante.

Stew a dozen shallots in some butter until soft. Stir in some flour and let it brown; add the juice of a lemon, ¼-pint of water, a clove, a teaspoonful of sugar, and a pinch of salt and pepper. Boil gently for a few minutes and stir in a little more flour; add ½-pt. of clear stock or water, boil for 15 minutes and strain.

160. Plain Brown Gravy.

Melt some butter until brown, add flour (previously mixed well in a little water), and some vegetable stock, dilute if necessary and strain. A fried onion and tomato, and a teaspoonful of Nutter adds to the flavour and richness. The addition of Vegeton, Nutril or Marmite improves this.

161. Sauce Piquante.

Take equal quantities of vegetable stock and Tomate à la Vatel (Dandicolle and Gaudin), fry a chopped onion brown, add the above, thicken with arrowroot, boil and strain.

162. Rich Brown Gravy.

Melt 1 oz. butter or nutter in a small saucepan, then add nearly a tablespoonful of flour, and keep stirring until you get a rich dark brown, being careful not to burn; now add slowly some stock made by stewing brown haricot beans, and simmer slowly for about 20 minutes. At serving time, add a good teaspoonful of Nutril, Wintox or Marmite.

163. Tarragon Sauce.

Melt 1-oz. of butter, stir in ½-oz. of flour until free from lumps, add ¼-pt. of milk and stir until it boils. Finally add 20 or 30 drops of Tarragon vinegar. This sauce is an excellent addition to cauliflower, and the flavour is unique.

164. Parsley Sauce.

Make in same way as in the above recipe, but substitute a large teaspoonful of finely chopped parsley for the vinegar.

165. Tomato Sauce.

Fry a sliced onion in butter until brown, add 6 sliced tomatoes, a clove of garlic and ½-oz. more butter. Heat until quite soft, add ½-pt. of clear vegetable stock or water, strain and serve. Thicken with arrowroot if desired.

166. Sauce Hollandaise.

Take 3-ozs. of butter, the juice of a lemon, the yolks of 3 eggs, and a teaspoonful of flour. Heat in a double saucepan while being stirred, until it begins to thicken. This is a good sauce to serve with cauliflower, asparagus, artichokes, etc.

167. White Sauce.

Make in the same manner as Tarragon Sauce, but omit the vinegar and add ¼-pt. of water.

168. Mayonnaise Sauce.

Mix a teaspoonful of mustard with the yolk of an egg, add 4 tablespoons of pure olive oil, a few drops at a time, beating it with a fork; add 2-ozs. of castor sugar, some pepper and salt, the juice of a large lemon and 2 teaspoons of Tarragon vinegar. Whisk the white of the egg with ¼-pint of cream, and beat all together.

169. Tomato Chutney.

One and a half pounds of tomatoes, 1-¾-lb. apples, 1½-lb. sultanas, 1½-lb. brown sugar, 2-ozs. onions, 4-ozs. salt, ¾-oz. cayenne pepper, 3-pts. vinegar. The whole to be boiled for 3 hours. Pour into stoppered bottles. This makes a most excellent chutney.

170. Coconut Sauce.

Melt 1-oz. of butter in a pan, stir in 1-oz. of flour smoothly, then add ½-pt. of cold water and ½-pt. of milk, half at a time; stir in ½-oz. of desiccated coconut and ½-oz. of sugar, and bring to the boil. Mapleton's Coconut Cream is superior to butter.

171. Marmite Savoury Gravy.

Chop an onion, and put it into 1-pt. of boiling water with a teaspoon of butter and a dessertspoon of dried sage; boil until the onion is soft; add two teaspoons of Marmite, season with pepper and salt, and thicken with a small teacupful of arrowroot or cornflour. Strain and serve.

172. Marmite Glaze.

Dissolve two teaspoons of Marmite in ½-pt. of boiling water, strain through a fine hair sieve or a piece of muslin into an enamel saucepan, put in 2-ozs. of gelatine, place on the fire and dissolve.

173. Quick Lunch Gravy.

Put a teaspoon of Marmite into a pint of boiling water, season with pepper and salt, thicken with a little browned flour.

174. Thick Brown Sauce.

Fry 1 onion, 1 lump of sugar, and a little butter until quite brown, add 2 teaspoons of brown flour and ½-pt. vegetable stock, pepper and salt to taste, boil well, and strain.

175. Carnos Sauce.

A Sauce can be quickly made with a spoonful of Carnos, thickened with flour, and flavoured to taste, with onion, tomato, or celery, etc.

176. Cheese Sauce.

Place ½-pt. of milk in a pan, and add a teaspoon of cornflour. Boil up and beat in 3-ozs. of grated cheese after removing from fire.

177. Fruit Sauce.

Take 1-oz. of cornflour, mix with a little water, adding ½-pt. of cherry, pineapple, or other fruit syrup, and boil until it thickens.

PUDDINGS AND SWEETS.

178. Christmas Pudding.

Mix 1-lb. breadcrumbs, 1-lb. flour, 1-lb. sultanas or currants, 2-lbs. raisins, ¼-lb. mixed peel, ½-lb. sugar, ½-lb. Nutter ((or Vegsu), flaked in the nut mill), ½-lb. chopped pine kernels. Add nutmeg to taste, and five or six eggs. Boil for 12 hours, and serve with sauce as usual. This pudding wins approbation from all who try it.

N.B.—All boiled puddings should be allowed ample room to swell during cooking. If too closely confined they are sometimes prevented from being light.

179. A Simple Plum Pudding.

Mix ½-lb. flour, 1-lb. raisins or sultanas, 6-ozs. Nutter and 1-oz. mixed peel. Add 1 teaspoonful of mixed spice, 2 eggs, and a little milk if required. Boil for at least 6 hours, serve with sweet sauce.

180. A Fruit Salad.

By the *Chef* of the Canton Hotel.

Peaches, apricots, cherries, grapes, black and red currants, pineapples, bananas. The peaches and apricots are peeled and quartered, the cherries stoned, the bananas and pineapples cut in slices or dice. Mix, cover with powdered sugar, a glass of kirsch, and a glass of maraschino, and lay on ice until required.

181. Rich Plum Pudding.

Take ½-lb. stoned raisins, ½-lb. sultanas, 2-ozs. mixed peel, ¼-lb. sugar, 4-ozs. breadcrumbs, ½-lb. chopped apples, 2-ozs. Nutter, 2-ozs. pine kernels, 6 sweet almonds, 6 Brazil nuts, ½ nutmeg, 2 teaspoons of mixed spice, 1 teaspoon of ginger, a few drops of ratafia flavouring essence, and 3 eggs. Finely chop all the fruit and the pine kernels, and put the nuts and peel through the mill. Rub the Nutter into the breadcrumbs and mix in the other ingredients and finally the eggs, one at a time (stirring well). Put into basins and boil 12 hours, then set aside till wanted. Boil them again for 2 or 3 hours before serving.

182. Sultana and Ginger Pudding.

Thoroughly mix 7-ozs. breadcrumbs, 1 oz. of flour, 8-ozs. sultanas, 3-ozs. sugar, and one good teaspoonful of ground ginger. Rub in 1-oz. butter and then stir in gradually 3 gills of milk and water (mixed), and lastly put in a small teaspoonful of carbonate of soda. Stir well, pour into a buttered mould and steam for three hours.

Chopped figs, French plums or dates can be substituted for the sultanas, and thus the pudding can be made in various ways.

183. Plain Sultana Pudding.

Mix in a basin 7-ozs. breadcrumbs, 1-oz. flour, 6-ozs. sultanas, 3-ozs. sugar, and 1-oz. butter. Moisten with ¾-pint of milk and water, to which has been added 1 small teaspoon of bicarbonate of soda. Steam for 3 hours, and serve with sweet sauce. This pudding is much appreciated by children.

184. Jellied Figs.

Stew ½-lb. of figs in 1-pt. of water for 2 or 3 hours till quite tender. Dissolve ½-oz. of gelatine in ½-pt. of water over a gentle heat and strain it on to the figs after they have been cut into small pieces and the juice of half a lemon added; stir well and turn into a wetted mould. Turn out when cold and sprinkle a little ground almond or coconut over it. Serve plain or with cream.

185. Creamed Rice Moulds.

Put 3-ozs. of rice into a saucepan with 1½-pts. of cold milk, bring to the boil, then stand over a gentle heat till quite tender, stirring occasionally to keep it from burning. Add vanilla, 1-oz. of sugar and ¼-pt. of cream, mix well and pour into wetted moulds. Serve garnished with raspberry or other jam.

186. Ambrosia.

Pare 5 oranges, removing all the tough white skin, cut through twice and slice them. Take a cup of grated coconut and moisten with cream. Fill a glass bowl with alternate layers of orange and coconut, finish with orange and cover with a thick layer of whipped cream, sprinkle with ground almonds, and decorate with candied fruit.

187. Bread Pudding.

Any piece of stale bread or cake, 3-ozs. sultanas, 3-ozs. currants, a little peel and spice, 1 egg, and sugar to taste. Soak the bread by pouring some boiling milk over it, beat it up very well, then add the fruit, etc., and bake or boil for 2 hours.

188. Semolina Moulds.

Cook 3-ozs. of semolina in 1½-pts of milk for three-quarters of an hour, stirring well, flavour with sugar and vanilla or lemon essence, and pour into wetted moulds. Serve with preserve garnishing.

189. Castle Puddings.

The weight of 2 eggs in butter and sugar, the weight of 3 eggs in flour and a little grated lemon rind. Cream the butter and sugar together, add the eggs well beaten and lemon rind. Mix well and stir in the flour, half fill the pudding moulds with the mixture and bake for 20 minutes. Serve with a jam sauce.

190. Strawberry Cream.

Half-pound strawberries, 3-ozs. castor sugar, 1 gill cream, ½-oz. gelatine, 2 eggs. Mash the strawberries to a pulp with the sugar, then add the cream, the yolks of eggs, and gelatine (dissolved in a little water) and cook over a saucepan of boiling water for 15 minutes, stirring all the time. Whip the whites of egg to a stiff froth and add to the mixture and cook for a few minutes more, then pour into a buttered mould, and turn out when stiff.

191. Marmalade Pudding.

Three-ozs. nut-margarine, 3-ozs. castor sugar, 2 tablespoons marmalade, 2 eggs, 6-ozs. flour. Beat the butter and sugar to a cream, then add the eggs and marmalade and beat well for 10 minutes, then stir in the flour very lightly, and put in a greased basin, cover with a greased paper and steam for 2 hours. Serve with sweet sauce.

192. Small Cakes.

Three-ozs. nut-margarine, 3-ozs. castor sugar, 2 eggs, 5-ozs. flour. Cream the butter and sugar together and add the eggs well beaten and stir the flour in lightly, mix well and put in a shallow tin and bake for 20 minutes. When cold cut in small shapes and ice.

193. Stewed Prunes à la Francaise.

Put the prunes in a basin of water and leave to soak for 12 hours, then stew gently in a double saucepan in the same water (with a slice of lemon peel) until it forms into a thick juice. Serve with whipped cream or boiled rice, etc.

194. Custard Moulds.

Boil 1-pt. milk with 1 tablespoonful sugar and 1 bay leaf; add ½-oz. gelatine. Stir till dissolved, and remove from the fire for a minute or two. Strain this on to 1 egg well beaten, return to pan, and stir over the fire until it thickens, but do not let it boil. Whisk well occasionally while cooling, and just before it sets pour into wetted moulds.

195. Bakewell Pudding.

Line a pie dish with puff paste, and spread on it a layer of apricot jam. Put the yolks of 2 eggs into a basin with the white of 1 and beat well together. Then add 3-ozs. of sugar, 2-ozs. butter dissolved, and ½-oz. of ground almonds. Mix all well together and pour over the jam; bake half-an-hour.

196. Vanilla Creams.

Dissolve ½-oz. of gelatine in 3 gills of milk, and flavour with 1-oz. of sugar and 1 teaspoonful of vanilla essence. Strain it on to ¼-pt. of cream, and when just beginning to set, whisk well and stir in lightly the white of an egg beaten till quite stiff. Turn into wetted moulds and leave till set.

197. Lemon Creams.

Dissolve ½-oz. of gelatine in ½-pt. of water, with 2-ozs. of sugar and the grated rind and juice of a lemon. When nearly cold strain this on to 1 gill of milk and 1 gill of cream, whisk well and stir in lightly the stiff-beaten white of an egg. Pour into moulds and leave till set.

198. Lemon Semolina Pudding.

Put three tablespoonfuls semolina in a saucepan with 1½-pts. milk. Bring to the boil, then simmer slowly till quite swollen. Set aside to cool a little, then add 2-ozs. sugar, the grated rind and half the juice of a lemon, also a well-beaten egg. Stir well and pour into a buttered pie-dish, and bake slowly till set. Turn out and garnish with jam.

199. Raspberry Pudding.

Stew 1-lb. of raspberries (or more) with some sugar. Line a basin with some slices of bread (without crust). Pour in half the fruit, cover with a layer of bread, then add the remainder of the raspberries and another layer of bread. Press down with a saucer and place a weight on it. Turn out and serve when cold with cream or Plasmon snow-cream.

200. Rice à la Reine.

Cook 3-ozs. rice in 1-qt. milk for 2 or 3 hours, sweeten and flavour to taste. When cooled a little add ½-oz. gelatine dissolved in ½-a-teacup of milk and strained, and 1 gill of cream; stir well and pour into a wetted mould.

201. Apple Custard.

Place some biscuit crumbs in a buttered pie dish. Nearly fill it with stewed apples. Beat an egg with ¼-pt. of milk and pour over the apples. Place some small ratafia biscuits on the top and some grated nutmeg. Bake in a moderate oven.

202. Sultana Custard Pudding.

To 2-ozs. of Robinson's Patent Barley, add 1-oz. of sifted sugar, ½-oz. of butter, a pinch of salt, and nearly 1-pt. of milk; mix thoroughly and stir it over the fire till it boils; then add a yolks of eggs, 3-ozs. sultanas, and bake the pudding in a buttered pie-dish.

203. Swiss Roll.

Take 3-ozs. castor sugar and 1 teacupful flour, and add to them 1 teaspoonful of baking powder. Separate the yolks from the whites of 2 eggs, and beat the latter till stiff. Add 1 tablespoon of milk to the yolks, and work into the flour and sugar, then add the stiffly beaten whites. Beat all well with a wooden spoon. Pour on to a greased Yorkshire pudding tin, and bake in a very hot oven for seven minutes. Then turn on to a piece of kitchen paper dredged with castor sugar. Spread quickly with jam (which has been thoroughly beaten) and roll with the paper. Place on a sieve till cool.

204. Gateau aux Fruits.

Take half a tinned pineapple, 3 bananas, ¼-lb. grapes, 4 Tangarine oranges, and the juice of a lemon. Cut up the fruit into dice, sprinkle with sugar and pour over them half the pineapple syrup, the lemon juice, and a tablespoonful of maraschino, and leave for an hour to soak. Split five stale sponge cakes open, cut each half into three fingers and spread each rather thickly with apricot jam. Place four of these strips on a glass dish so as to form a square, and put four more across the corners so as to form a diamond in it, and so on, square and diamond alternately. Fill the middle of the tower thus formed with the macedoine of fruits, piling them high above the top, and pour the rest of the pineapple syrup over the cake. Whip half a pint of cream stiffly, and put it (or Coconut Cream, 224) on in rough spoonfuls all over the tower.

205. Poached Apricots.

Upon some slices of sponge cake, place half an apricot (round side uppermost). Whip some white of egg to a snow frost with castor sugar. Place this round the apricot so as to make it resemble a poached egg. Whipped cream is preferable to many persons if obtainable. The sponge should be slightly moistened with the apricot juice.

206. Lemon Sponge.

Dissolve ½-oz. of leaf gelatine in ½-pt. of water and add the rind of a lemon and 1-oz. castor sugar. Strain the juice of a lemon on to the white of an egg, then strain the dissolved gelatine on to it. Whisk all together till it makes quite a stiff froth. Turn into a mould, and take out when set.

207. Plasmon Snow-Cream.

Put 3 heaped teaspoonfuls (1-¾-ozs.) of Plasmon into a bowl. From ½-pt. of tepid water take 4 tablespoons and mix it with the powder, rubbing it into a paste. Slowly add the remainder of the water; stir thoroughly, then place in a saucepan and bring to the boil, stirring all the time. Stand aside to get quite cold. When required for use, whisk it into a thick snow-cream. This makes a splendid addition to stewed fruit (peaches, &c.), cocoa, coffee, or puddings. It is most nutritious also. The proportions must be correct to get the cream *firm* as well as *light*. If it is *frothy* there is too much water; if sticky and heavy there is not sufficient water.

208. Rice and Sultana Padding.

To an ordinary rice pudding add 4-ozs. of sultanas. Bake in a slow oven for several hours, with plenty of milk. When cooked it should be brown in colour and quite moist. It is easily digested and makes a good supper dish.

209. Plain Boiled Pudding.

Take 2-ozs. of Nutter, 4-ozs. each of white and brown flour, and 4-ozs. of breadcrumbs. Add water gradually, mixing into a dry dough, and boil in a cloth for an hour and a half.

210. Apple Fritters.

Peel and quarter, or finely mince, some good cooking apples, dip in batter made as follows:—1 tablespoonful flour, 1 egg well beaten, enough milk to make it the consistency of cream. Fry crisp, and serve.

211. Empress Pudding.

Take 1-pt. of breadcrumbs, 1-qt. of new milk, the yolks of 4 eggs (well beaten), the grated rind of a lemon, and 3-ozs. of butter; mix and bake about half an hour. When cold, spread some raspberry or plum jam over the pudding, then whip the whites of the eggs with a teacup of sifted sugar and the juice of a lemon, and lay this over the jam. Make slightly brown in the oven.

212. Orange Jelly.

Wipe and thickly peel 5 oranges and 2 lemons, take 1-pt. of cold water, ½-lb. white sugar, and 1½-ozs. cornflour. Place the peel and water in a pan and simmer for 20 minutes with the sugar; strain the resulting juice. Place the cornflour in a basin and squeeze the juice of the fruit through a strainer on to it, then pour the boiling syrup on to this mixture; stir well, return to saucepan, and boil for 6 minutes. Pour out into cold wet mould. Garnish with orange.

213. Ginger Pudding.

Take 6-ozs. of brown breadcrumbs (finely grated), 3-ozs. of butter, a saltspoonful of ground ginger, the juice of a lemon, and 4-ozs. of castor sugar. Stir these in a stewpan until the butter is melted. Chop 4-ozs. of preserved ginger and add to the mixture with the yolks of 2 eggs. Beat well together and set aside to cool. Whisk the whites of the eggs and stir into the pudding quickly. Fill a buttered basin with it, cover with a saucer (leaving room to swell) and steam for 3 hours. Serve with cream or fruit sauce (177).

214. Baked Coconut Custard.

Beat 3 eggs and mix with 1½-pts. of milk, add 2 tablespoons of desiccated coconut, and a tablespoonful of sugar. Bake in a slow oven, and add some grated nutmeg.

215. Semolina Pudding.

Boil a teacupful of semolina for 15 minutes in 2½ pts. of milk, stirring all the time. Flavour with vanilla. Turn out into a buttered pie dish, garnish with ratafia biscuits and bake in a moderate oven.

216. Strawberry Cream Ice.

Take 1½-lbs. of ripe strawberries, 6-ozs. of castor sugar, ½-lb. of cream and a teacupful of milk. Put the strawberries through a sieve or strainer, mix the whole well together, and freeze.

Raspberry ice can be made in a simpler form by reducing the cream by one-half and by adding another teacupful of milk in which a dessertspoonful of cornflour has been boiled.

217. Vanilla Ice.

Take 1 pint of milk, 1 gill of cream, the yolks of 3 eggs, and 3-ozs. of castor sugar. After heating the milk, mix ½-oz. of ground rice with a little cold milk and put it in the saucepan. Pour in the beaten yolks and cream, and the sugar; stir and simmer until the custard thickens, strain and set aside to cool; add vanilla to taste, and stir well; place in the freezing machine. To make this ice taste richer and more delicate, reduce the milk and increase the cream.

218. Lemon Cheese-Cakes.

Put in a saucepan ¼-lb. butter, 1-lb. lump sugar, 6 eggs (leaving out 2 whites), 2 grated lemon rinds, and the juice of 3 lemons. Simmer until all is dissolved (gently stirring), and add a few dry biscuit crumbs. Serve on crisp pastry.

219. Lemon Jelly.

Dissolve 1-oz. of isinglass in 1-¼-pts. of water. Add the grated peel of 2 lemons and ½-lb. of lump sugar. Boil for 10 minutes, stirring continually. Take off fire and add the juice of 1½ lemons. Strain and cool. Whisk well before turning into moulds.

220. Fruitarian Mincemeat.

Take 7-ozs. Nutter, 12-ozs. raisins, 6-ozs. sultanas, 6-ozs. currants, ¼-lb. Demerara sugar, 1½-lbs. apples, ¼-lb. mixed candied peel, the rind and juice of 1 lemon, 6 almonds, 6 Brazil nuts, a few drops ratafia flavouring essence, and 3 teaspoons of mixed spice. Stone the rasins, finely chop all the fruit, and put the nuts and almonds through the nut mill. Now melt the Nutter in a saucepan, and gradually add all the other ingredients, stirring well, leave standing over night, and put in pots next morning. Cover closely, and this will keep a long time.

221. Short Pastry.

Rub ½-lb. Nutter into 1-lb. flour and 2-ozs. Artox wholemeal, mix as dry as possible with water, and it is ready to make excellent biscuits, short cakes, or tart crusts. If whiter pastry is required use white flour.

222. Puff Pastry.

Ingredients:—1-lb. flour, ¾-lb. Nutter, cold water. Method:—Rub ¼-lb. Nutter into the flour, mix to a rough dough with cold water, stand in a cool place for ten minutes. Roll out and "spot" over with ¼-lb. Nutter broken in small pieces; fold over, roll out and stand 10 minutes. Roll out again and spot over with the remaining ¼-lb. Nutter; fold over and roll out, and after standing 10 minutes it is ready for use.

223. Chestnut Cream.

Take from 20 to 30 chestnuts, remove the shells and skins. Put the chestnuts in a saucepan with 2 teacups full of water, sugar to taste, the juice of 1 lemon, and simmer slowly until they are quite soft. Pass through a sieve or potato masher, and when cold pile in a dish, and cover with whipped cream.

224. Coconut Cream.

A nice addition to Trifles, Fruit Salads, etc., can be made by using Mapleton's Coconut Cream. Mix 2 ozs. of the cream with 1/8-pt. of boiling water; when softened beat for a minute or so with the egg-beater, then pour on a dish. In 2 hours it will have set and can be used to fill sponge sandwiches, or eaten with stewed fruit. To form a thick cream (less solid) beat up 2½ to 3 ozs. Coconut Cream with ¼-pt. of hot water.

THE BREAD PROBLEM.

Pure wholemeal bread, so made as to be light and well baked, is a virtual necessity for every abstainer from flesh-food. Food-Reform presents many difficulties, and every dietetic reformer has to grapple with them. Insufficient knowledge, defective sources of provision, digestive troubles, inherited organic weakness, and unfavourable environment, are only a few of these. I want, therefore to emphasize the importance of a perfect bread supply, which I am convinced is the key to the problem so far as many are concerned.

It is not sufficient merely to pray for "our daily bread," and then to leave its provision entirely to Providence. We need also to *think* and to take some personal trouble about it—remembering that Heaven helps those who help themselves. Yet this is what very few people do. One may safely affirm that four persons out of every five are content to use defective and innutritious bread every day of their lives. Yet this should be made a real staff of life.

The whole grain of wheat, if of good quality, contains nearly all that is needful for the perfect nutrition of the body. With the addition of a small amount of fat (easily found in nut or dairy butter, cheese or oil), and of grape sugar and purifying acids (obtainable in fruits), pure wheatmeal, if properly ground in stone mills, and well made into delicious home-baked bread, enables one to be almost independent of other foods, and therefore almost ensures one against a breakdown in health if there is difficulty in obtaining a varied and well proportioned dietary from other sources.

Instead of securing and using bread such as this, the majority of the community complacently eat white bread—emasculated, robbed of its gluten (which is equivalent to albumen) and of the phosphates and mineral salts that are stored in the inner part of the husk of the grain. It is composed almost entirely of starch, with the addition of such adulterants as the baker or miller feels inclined to introduce for commercial reasons, and is not conducive to the proper operation of the digestive and eliminative organs.

It is difficult for bakers or the public to buy really good wholemeal. The meal that is on the markets often consists of cheap roller-milled flour with some sweepings of bran or seconds thrown in. And even if the entire grain is supplied, the outer cuticle of the wheat, when *rolled* (in the modern steel-roller mills that for reasons of economy have superseded the good old-fashioned stone *grinding* mills), instead of being so reduced as to be capable of complete digestion, is left with rough edges called *spiculae*, which irritate the digestive tract, cause relaxation, and arouse prejudice against the 'brown' loaf. Such wholemeal cannot be perfectly assimilated because the bran is not properly broken up, and, in addition to this fact, the cerealine, which acts like diastase in the conversion of starch into sugar, is not liberated and rendered available as an aid to digestion.

That the distasteful and often indigestible brown or wholemeal bread (so-called) usually sold by bakers is either defective or adulterated, can easily be proven by anyone. Let any reader procure some stone-milled entire wheatmeal that is guaranteed pure (I use the 'Artox' and 'Ixion' brands myself, because I believe them to be of genuine quality and properly stone-ground); then make some thin loaves as described in the following recipe. The result, if the bread is skilfully made, will be a delicious and nutritive loaf of the farmhouse type with a sweet nutty flavour. Instead of quickly getting 'stale,' such a loaf is enjoyable when four days old, and it only needs to be compared with ordinary bakers' bread to reveal the fact that it is an entirely different article of food. Its sustaining power is wonderful, and it proves an effectual preventive of starved nerves as well as other ailments.

225. How to make Wholemeal Bread.

The yeast must be quite fresh, and the bread should be raised in separate tins *in a warm place or cupboard*; the oven must be hot at first, but the heat should be much reduced after 10 minutes. Mix 6-lbs. of wholemeal with 1-lb. of household flour. Then mix 3-ozs. of *fresh* yeast with a tablespoon of treacle, adding 2 tablespoons of olive oil when it is quite dissolved. Put this into the flour with about 2-pts. of lukewarm water. Mix it with a wooden spoon till it does not stick. Knead for 10 minutes, adding more water if necessary but keeping the dough firm and spongy. Put it into flat baking tins (well greased) about 2½ inches deep, covering the tins to the depth of about 1 inch only. Let it rise for 1 hour, or till it reaches the tops of the tins. Then bake first in a quick oven, and afterwards in a slower. A gas oven is most reliable for baking bread, as the heat is more easily regulated. The bread should be a rich dark golden brown when well baked.

226. White Bread.

Make as Recipe 225, but substitute household flour for wholemeal. The shape and size of the loaves should be changed occasionally. Loaves baked in *small* tins are often lighter than bread made into large loaves.

227. Plain Currant Bread and Buns.

To 2-lbs. of good wholemeal or white flour add a pinch of salt, 1 tablespoonful of sugar, and ½-lb. of currants or sultanas; also rub in 2-ozs. of olive oil or nut-margarine. Mix 1-oz. of yeast with a little golden syrup and add lukewarm water. Stir this into the flour, and add sufficient warm water to make a nice dough. Shape into loaves or little buns, set to rise for 1 hour or longer, then bake in a quick oven and brush with egg and milk.

228. Dinner Rolls.

Delicious dinner rolls can be made as follows:—Take 1-lb. of white flour, 1-lb. of wholemeal, 3-ozs. butter, and 1-oz. of yeast. Mix the yeast with a dessertspoonful of treacle, ¾-pt. of milk and water. Rub the butter into the flour, and put in the yeast to rise. Knead, form into small rolls, raise for half-an-hour, bake in a quick oven.

229. Sultana Cake.

Sift into ½-lb. of flour 1 teaspoonful of baking powder. Grate the rind of a lemon on to an egg and beat it well. Cream together 3-ozs. nut-margarine and 3-ozs. sugar; add the egg, beating still, then stir in lightly the flour and 3-ozs. sultanas; add milk to make a soft dough. Pour into a well-buttered cake tin, put in a hot oven, and bake for about half-an-hour, reducing the temperature considerably.

230. Sultana Rice Cake.

Put 3-ozs. of Nut-margarine in a warm oven. Grate the rind of a lemon on to an egg and 3-ozs. of castor sugar, beat well, then add the warmed Nutter and beat again till it is creamy. Now sift together 5-ozs. of ground rice, 3-ozs. of flour and 1 teaspoonful of baking powder. Beat this gently into the mixture, add 4-ozs. sultanas and enough milk to make a proper consistency. Put in a hot oven, gradually reducing the temperature, and bake for about ¾ of an hour.

231. Cheese Straws.

Mix 6-ozs. flour and 6-ozs. grated cheese well together, then rub in 2-ozs. butter, add a little cayenne pepper and salt, bind with the yolk of an egg, roll out about a quarter of a inch thick, cut into long narrow fingers, and bake in a sharp oven for 10 minutes.

232. Sultana Bun Cakes.

Sift together 8-ozs. of flour, 3-ozs. Paisley flour and 2-ozs. of sugar; rub in 4-ozs. olive oil, and add 4-ozs. of sultanas. Mix all with a well beaten egg and a little milk, roll out, shape with a cutter and bake at once in a quick oven.

SUMMER AND WINTER DRINKS.

The following recipes and suggestions concerning a few beverages which can be used as substitutes for more stimulating drinks may prove useful to many readers:—

233. Barley Water.

Mix a tablespoonful of Pearl Barley with a pint of water and boil for half-an-hour. Flavour with lemon, cinnamon or sugar, according to taste, and allow the mixture to cool. For invalids requiring nutriment a larger quantity of barley should be used.

Barley Water is equally suitable for winter use and can be taken hot.

234. Wheatenade.

Simmer 1-lb. of crushed wheat in 1-qt. of water for about an hour, stirring it occasionally. Strain, add lemon juice and sugar to taste, for use in summer, or milk and sugar if the drink is taken hot in winter. Good and clean bran can be substituted for crushed wheat. This is a capital drink for children with a tendency to rickets, or for persons suffering from nervous prostration caused by malnutrition.

235. Oatenade.

Simmer ¼-lb. of coarse oatmeal in the same manner as described in the previous recipe, then flavour to taste. This drink will be slightly richer in fat than the previous one, and it makes a good winter drink.

236. Gingerade.

Take 1-dr. essence cayenne, 4-drs. essence of ginger, 2-drs. essence of lemon, 1-dr. burnt sugar, ¾-oz. of tartaric acid. Add 3-lbs. lump sugar and 5-qts. boiling water. Bottle ready for use. Dilute to taste.

237. Fruit Drink.

Lime juice, if pure, makes a cooling and wholesome drink. The "Montserrat" is one of the purest brands upon the market; some of the liquid sold as lime juice is only a chemical concoction. The weaker the solution the better it tastes. A dessertspoonful to the tumbler is generally enough. Dole's Pineapple juice is also an excellent fruit drink.

238. Rice Water.

Boil some once-milled rice in water, and add lemon juice and sugar to taste. The beverage should not be made too thick. As rice is often used in most households a supply of this nutritious drink is easily provided. It is very good for children.

Tea and Coffee Substitutes.

Those who find tea and coffee undesirable should try "Wallace P. R. Coffee," "Lifebelt Coffee," "Salfon," or "Horlick's Malted Milk." Another good substitute is "Hygiama," which, unlike tea and coffee, is not a stimulant, but a nutrient. On the other hand its effect on the system is distinctly stimulating in a right and healthy sense. That is to say, the valuable nourishment which it contains is very easily and quickly digested and an immediate sense of invigoration is the result. Unlike cocoa, it is not clogging or constipating or heavy.

HOW TO FEED INVALIDS.

In all cases of sickness the patient will have a better chance of recovery if the diet is light and wisely selected.

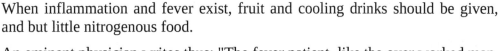

When inflammation and fever exist, fruit and cooling drinks should be given, and but little nitrogenous food.

An eminent physician writes thus: "The fever patient, like the over worked man, digests badly. He has no appetite; his salivary glands do not secrete, or secrete very imperfectly. The gastric juice formed under bad conditions is almost inert, poor in pepsine and hydrocloric acid. The liver no longer acts if the fever is high and serious; the intestinal secretions are partially exhausted.... The fever patient must then be fed very little."

When the hydrocloric acid is deficient, proteid food should be given very sparingly—one of the best forms being Casumen in solution (see 224) or white of egg. Milk is not advisable in such a condition, unless malted, or in the dried form. Fats are objectionable, and if the salivary secretions are defective, starches should be given in dextrinized (super-cooked) form, or well toasted. Fruit sugars, which are Carbohydrates in a digested form, are better still, and may be given freely to patients of nearly all kinds. They are abundantly provided in figs, dates, stoneless raisins and sultanas, and in other sweet fruits, such as bananas, strawberries and apples.

Ample nourishment can be provided by these, supplemented by egg dishes (chiefly white); flaked and super-cooked cereals, such as Granose Biscuits, Kellogg Wheat Flakes, Wallace P. R. and Flakit Biscuits, Archeva Rusks, Melarvi Crisps, and toasted or wholemeal bread; flaked or malted nuts; legumes soufflé; well-cooked farinaceous puddings; Horlick's Malted Milk and many other proprietary health-foods; and vegetable broths—for which see Recipes 1-23, as well as those which conclude this section on pages 123 and 124.

One of the most important of these latter is 'Haricot Broth,' which is a perfect substitute for "beef tea," being far more nutritious and also free from the toxic elements which are contained in that dangerous and superstitiously venerated compound.

The Beef Tea Delusion. Dr. Milner Fothergill stated that probably more invalids have sunk into their graves through a misplaced confidence in the value of beef tea than Napoleon killed in all his wars. It is, in reality, a strong solution of waste products and of uric acid, consisting largely of excrementitious matter which was in process of elimination from the system of some animal, through the minute drain pipes which form an important cleansing medium or "sewage system" in all animal flesh. To make "beef tea," these poisonous substances are stewed out to form the decoction, while the animal fibrin, the portion of the meat that has some nutritive value, is thrown away.

Beef tea consequently acts as a strong stimulant, tends to increase inflammation and fever, and in all such cases lessens the chance of the patient's recovery, as the system is already battling against toxic elements in the blood. To add to the amount of the latter is obviously unwise and dangerous. These remarks apply also to 'meat essences' and to 'beef extracts,' which are frequently made from diseased flesh which has been condemned in the slaughterhouses.

Meals provided for invalids should be very simple, but served in a very dainty manner. A spotless serviette and tray cloth, bright silver, a bunch of flowers and a ribbon to match them in colour for tying the serviette (the colour of which can be changed from day to day) should not be forgotten. The food should be supplied in small quantities; half a cupful of broth will often be taken when a cupful would be sent away untouched, and the wishes of the patient should be respected so far as it is safe and wise to do so. It is also a good plan to serve two or three small separate courses, rather than to put everything that is provided on a tray together.

Stewed French plums and figs are valuable in the sickroom because of their laxative effects, and dainty sandwiches will be found acceptable by most invalids—made with flaked nuts and honey, dried milk (Lacvitum), potted meat, etc.

Don't Overfeed Invalids. One of the greatest evils to be avoided by those who are nursing the sick is that of over-feeding. When nature is doing her best to meet a crisis, or to rid the body of microbes or impurities, it is a mistake to cause waste of vital energy by necessitating the expulsion of superfluous alimentary matter. Invalids should not be unduly persuaded to take food. The stomach generally requires *rest*, and is often in such a condition that digestion is impossible.

Much of the suffering and inconvenience endured by sick persons is simply the result of erroneous diet. Judicious feeding will do far more than drugs to alleviate and cure most maladies, in fact drugs and stimulants are seldom required. The great healing agent is the Life-force within—the "*Vis medicatrix Naturæ*"—and the wise physician will see that this power has a fair chance. He will encourage hopeful mental influence, and advocate pure air, pure food, and pure water, combined with a cessation of any physical transgression which has been the *cause* of the malady in question.

Care should be exercised lest invalids partake too freely of starch foods, especially if such are insufficiently cooked. Wholemeal bread should be *light* and *well baked*, and in most cases it will be more easily assimilated if toasted. Granose and other similar biscuits (which consist of entire wheatmeal in a super-cooked form, so that the starch is already transformed into 'dextrin') will be easily digestible and are slightly laxative in their effect. They are just the right thing to be taken with broth or soup or porridge. The following recipes will be found helpful.

239. Brown Haricot Broth.

(A perfect substitute for 'Beef Tea.')

Take ½-lb. of brown haricot beans. Wash and stew them with 1-qt. of hot water and some small onions for 3 hours, stewing down to 1-pt. Strain, and add pepper, celery-salt and butter when serving. This bean tea or broth, so prepared, will be found to be very savoury and of the same taste and appearance as beef tea, while being much richer in nutriment.

240. Mock Chicken Broth.

A valuable substitute for chicken broth, which is in every way superior to the decoction obtained by stewing the flesh and bones of the bird, can be made by stewing and serving white haricots in the same manner as in the previous recipe.

241. Hygiama Apple Purée.

Select two or three sound ripe apples, wash and rub in hot water, remove core and all bruised or dark parts, but not the peel, cut in small pieces, place in a covered jar or casserole with a cupful of water, or sufficient to prevent burning. Cook gently until apples are soft; then rub all through a fine sieve. Mix a tablespoonful or more of Hygiama with just enough water to form a paste, mix this paste into the apple, with just a touch of cinnamon or nutmeg if liked, and serve with pieces of dry toast, twice-baked bread or rusks.

242. Oat Cream.

A most excellent recipe for invalids and anæmic patients is prescribed by Dr. Oldfield, as follows: Boil 1 pint milk, sift into it a large handful of crushed oats. Simmer until it is thick as raw cream. Strain and serve; the patient to take ½-pint, sucking it through a straw slowly.

243. Linseed Tea.

Few persons realize the good qualities of linseed tea. It is useful for weak, anæmic and delicate persons; it produces flesh, is soothing in bronchial cases, and laxative. If made thin, and flavoured with lemon, it is quite palatable, and many persons get fond of it. The seed should be whole and of best quality, and it only requires stewing until the liquor is of the consistency of thin gruel.

244. proteid Gruel.

A good liquid food can be quickly made by warming a dessertspoonful of "Emprote" or "Malted Nuts" in a glass of milk, and flavouring to taste. A large teaspoonful of "Casumen" (pure milk proteid) dissolved in a breakfastcup of barley water, coffee, or vegetable soup, also readily provides much nutriment in a simple form.

245. Lentil Gruel.

This is a useful and nutritious food for invalids. To make the gruel, take a dessertspoonful of lentil flour, mixed smooth in some cold milk, add nearly 1-pt. of milk which has been brought to the boil. Boil for 15 minutes and flavour with a little cinnamon or vanilla. Serve with toast. This is the same as the much prescribed "Revalenta Arabica" food, but the lentil flour, without a long scientific name, only costs 3d. a pound, instead of half-a-crown.

246. Malted Milk Prune Whip.

One cup of prunes, 2 tablespoonfuls Horlick's Malted Milk, 1 tablespoonful sugar, lemon sufficient to flavour, white of egg. Wash well, and soak the prunes until tender. Boil with small piece of lemon until soft. Add sugar, remove stones, rub through colander; add the Horlick's Malted Milk, beat well; add the white of egg, well beaten. Cool, and serve with whipped cream. Flavour with vanilla if desired.

247. Malted Milk Jelly.

Phosphated gelatine 1 teaspoonful, Horlick's Malted Milk 2 to 4 teaspoonfuls, sugar and flavouring to suit. Soak the gelatine in cold water for 1 hour, then dissolve in just sufficient hot water. Add the Horlick's Malted Milk dissolved in 2 cups of hot water, and sweeten and flavour to taste.

248. Malted Milk with Iced Fruit.

Take of Horlick's Malted Milk 1 heaped teaspoonful, crushed fruit 1 tablespoonful, crushed ice 1 tablespoonful, 1 egg, acid phosphate twenty drops, grated nutmeg to flavour, water to make a cup. Mix the Malted Milk, crushed fruit and egg, beating the same for five minutes. Add the phosphate and crushed ice, stirring all for several minutes. Strain, and add ice-cold water or cold carbonated water, and grated nutmeg to flavour.

249. Effervescent Malted Milk.

Put some finely cracked ice into a glass. Fill it half full of soda, Vichy or Syphon water, and immediately add the desired amount of Horlick's Malted Milk in solution. Drink while effervescing. Brandy may be added if necessary.

WHAT TO DO AT CHRISTMAS.

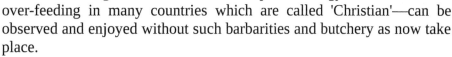

The Christmas festival—which has degenerated into such a deplorable orgy of massacre and over-feeding in many countries which are called 'Christian'—can be observed and enjoyed without such barbarities and butchery as now take place.

How can we consistently sing and talk of 'Peace on Earth' when we are participating in ruthless warfare against the animal creation?

Is not this wholesale and cruel slaughter altogether discordant with the spirit and doctrine of the gentle and harmless Teacher of Nazareth, whose terrestrial birth is thus celebrated by pagan barbarity? Should not those of us who dare to call ourselves His followers protest against a custom which brings discredit upon His religion and causes humanely disposed Oriental nations to regard it almost with contempt?

The following suggestive Menu will at once show my readers that Christmas can be celebrated with a feast of good things without such butchery. And many are they who have found that its joys can even be enhanced by a sense of freedom from blood-guiltiness and personal responsibility concerning the deeds that are done in the shambles at this time of 'Peace and Goodwill.'

The Menu can be varied as taste and circumstances may dictate.

A Bloodless Menu for Christmas.

From which a selection can be made.

Mock Turtle Soup (4).
Fried Bread Dice.

Julienne Soup (9).
Granose Biscuits.

Mock Scallop Oysters (24).

Mock White Fish (32).
Parsley Sauce.

Savoury Nut Steaks (50).

Macaroni Rissoles (68).
Sauce Piquante.

Yorkshire Pudding.

Potato Purée (109).

Cauliflowers.

Baked Stuffed Tomatoes (104).

Chestnut or Vegetable Soufflé (94 or 97).

Plum Pudding (178).

Stewed Pears.
Clotted Cream.

Mince Pies (220).

Fresh Fruits.

Almonds and Muscatels.

Figs.

Dates.

Preserved Ginger.

The cost of such a dinner as this will be much less than that of a corresponding one which includes poultry, game, and joints of flesh. The amount saved could be appropriately expended in providing a few comforts for the poor and needy—thus the Christmas festival provides an opportunity for lessening the suffering in this world, and also for increasing the sum of human happiness.

MENUS FOR THE WEEK.

By MRS. WALTER CAREY.

The following Menus may be a guide to beginners, and show how easy it is to get variety:—

Breakfast Menu, No. 1.

Manhu Oats. Porridge. Tea or Coffee. Scrambled Eggs on Toast.
Grilled Tomatoes, No. 122. Neapolitan Sausages, No. 123.
Brown Bread. Honey. Marmalade. Butter. Fruit.

Breakfast Menu, No. 2.

Manhu Rye Porridge. Tea or Coffee. Granose Biscuits.
Eggs à la Crême, No. 84. Savoury Rissoles, No. 98. Brown Bread.
Honey. Jam. Butter. Fruit.

Breakfast Menu, No. 3.

Manhu Wheat Porridge. Tea or Coffee. Omelette aux Tomates, No. 82.
Potted White Haricots, No. 144. Stewed French Plums, No. 193.
Brown Bread. Honey. Jam. Butter. Fruit.

Breakfast Menu, No. 4.

Ixion Kornules. Tea or Coffee. Toast.
Omelette aux Fines Herbes, No. 87. Grilled Mushrooms.
Brown Bread. Baked Apples. Butter. Marmalade. Honey. Fruit.

Breakfast Menu, No. 5.

Manhu Barley Porridge. Tea or Coffee.
Baked Stuffed Tomatoes, No. 104. Marmite Toast, No. 128.
Stewed French Plums. Brown Bread. Butter. Marmalade.
Honey. Fruit.

Breakfast Menu, No. 6.

Granose Flakes with Hot Milk. Tea or Coffee. Savoury Rissoles, No. 98.
Scrambled Eggs and Tomatoes, No. 88. Brown Bread.
Stewed Apples. Butter. Marmalade. Honey. Fruit.

Breakfast Menu, No. 7.

Manhu Wheat Porridge. Tea or Coffee. Granose Biscuits.
Stewed Figs. Fried Eggs and Mushrooms. Milanese Croquettes, No. 113.
Brown Bread. Butter. Marmalade. Fruit.

Cold Luncheon Menu, No. 1.

Oeufs Farcie en Aspic, No. 131. Salad & Mayonnaise Dressing, No. 156.
Potted Meat Sandwiches, No. 152. Poached Apricots, No. 205.
Jellied Figs, No. 184. Milk Cheese, No. 155. Scotch Oat Cakes.
Coffee. Fruit.

Cold Luncheon Menu, No. 2.

Nut Galantine, No. 132. Salad and Mayonnaise Dressing, No. 156.
Egg and Cress Sandwiches, No. 148. Lemon Sponge, No. 206.
Stewed and Fresh Fruit. Camembert Cheese. Biscuits. Coffee.

Luncheon Menu, No. 3.

Mock Lobster Shapes in Aspic, No. 135. Tomato Salad.
Egg Sandwiches, No 147. Mock Chicken Rolls, No. 60.
Orange Jelly, No. 212. Creamed Rice Moulds, No. 185.
Gruyère Cheese. Biscuits. P. R. Crackers. Coffee. Fruit.

Luncheon Menu, No. 4.

White Haricot Soup, No. 13. Mock Scallop Oysters, No. 24.
Eggs Florentine, No. 83. Cheese Soufflé. Fruit Tart.
Custard. Cheese. Fruit. Coffee.

Luncheon Menu, No. 5.

Tomato Soup, No. 6. Mock White Fish, No. 32.
Walnut Cutlets, No. 34. Green Peas. Mashed Potatoes.
Castle Puddings, No. 189. Meringues. Cheese. Fruit. Coffee.

Luncheon Menu, No. 6.

Brazil Nut Soup, No. 8. Mock Oyster Patties, No. 25.
Chestnut Stew, No. 130. Creamed Macaroni, No. 70.
Rice and Sultana Pudding, No. 208. Apple Fritters, No. 210.
Cheese. Fruit. Coffee.

Luncheon Menu, No. 7.

Julienne Soup, No. 9. Mock White Fish, No. 32.
Savoury Golden Marbles, No. 116. Brown Sauce, No. 174.
French Beans. Stuffed Vegetable Marrow, No. 112.
Empress Pudding, No. 211. Cheese Straws. Fruit. Coffee.

Dinner Menu, No. 1.

Soups—Mock Turtle Soup, No. 4. Dinner Rolls, No. 228.
Fish—Fillets of Mock Sole, No. 29. Sauce Hollandaise, No. 166.
Rôti—Nut Timbale, No. 65. Spinach Soufflé, No. 92.
Potato Croquettes, No. 117.
Entrée—Macaroni à la Turque, No. 67.

Dinner Menu, No. 2.

Soup—Chestnut Soup, No. 2. Granose Biscuits. Dinner Rolls, No. 228.
Fish—Mock White Fish, No. 32.
Rôti—Mock Steak Pudding, No. 59. Parsley Sauce, No 164.
Green Peas. Potato Purée, No. 109.
Entrée—Spinach Soufflé, No. 92.
Sweets—Sultana and Ginger Pudding, No. 182. Cream, or
Fruit Sauce, No. 177. Jellied Figs, No. 184.
Dessert—Fruit. Salted Almonds, No. 129. Dry Ginger. Coffee.

Dinner Menu, No. 3.

Soup—Celery Soup, No. 16.
Fish—Omelet aux fine Herbes, No. 87.
Rôti—Chestnut and Mushroom Pudding, No. 59. Flaked Potatoes.
Brussels Sprouts Sauté, No. 102.
Entrée—Green Pea Soufflé, No. 93.
Sweets—Jam Roll. Stewed French Plums, No. 193.
Dessert—Fruit. Sultanas. Figs. Almonds. Coffee.

Dinner Menu, No. 4.

Soup—White Haricot Soup, No. 13. Croûtons.
Fish—Mock Oyster Patties, No. 25.
Rôti—Mock Sweetbread Quenelles, No. 43. Mashed Potatoes.
Cauliflower.
Entrée—Asparagus Soufflé, No. 96.
Sweets—Marmalade Pudding, No. 191. Vanilla Creams.
Dessert—Fruit. Dry Ginger. Biscuits. Coffee.

Dinner Menu, No. 5.

Soup—Green Lentil Soup, No. 10. Granose Biscuits.
Fish—Fried Chinese Artichokes, No. 27.
Rôti—Walnut Rissoles, No. 37. French Beans.
Mashed Potatoes, No. 109.
Entrée—Omelet, No. 81. Spinach à la Crême, No. 91.
Sweets—Apple Custard, No. 201. Lemon Cheese Cakes, No. 218.
Dessert—Dry Ginger. Dates. Fruit. Fancy Biscuits. Coffee.

Dinner Menu, No 6.

Soups—Tomato Soup, No. <u>6</u>. Fried Bread Dice.
Fish—Mock Scallop Oysters, No. <u>24</u>.
Rôti—Purée of Walnuts, No. <u>40</u>. Spinach à la Crême, No. <u>91</u>.
Mashed Potatoes, No. <u>109</u>.
Entrée—Macaroni Cutlets, No. <u>68</u>.
Sweets—Empress Pudding, No. <u>211</u>. Orange Jelly, No. <u>212</u>.
Dessert—Dry Ginger. Fruit. Fancy Biscuits. Figs and Dates.
Coffee.

Dinner Menu, No. 7.

Soup—Artichoke Soup, No. <u>1</u>. Granose Biscuits.
Fish—Green Artichokes, No. <u>26</u>.
Rôti—Nut Croquettes, No. <u>41</u>. Yorkshire Pudding, No. <u>119</u>.
Brown Gravy, No. <u>162</u>. Mashed Potatoes, No. <u>109</u>.
Entrée—Baked Stuffed Tomatoes, No. <u>104</u>.
Sweets—Fruit Salad, No. <u>180</u>. Custard Moulds, No. <u>194</u>.
Dessert—Fruit. Salted Almonds. Roast Pine Kernels.
Dry Ginger. Biscuits. Coffee.

Hints to Housekeepers.

A few simple hints to those who are trying the vegetarian recipes in this book may be useful.

Cooking utensils should be kept quite separate from those used for meat, fish or fowl.

Nut-oil or nut-butter should always be used for frying, and the right heat is known when a slight blue haze rises above the pan, or by dipping a finger of bread in the oil, when if hot enough it will at once fry brown and crisp. After frying it is always best to place the articles fried on some folded tissue paper to drain out the frying oil.

Marmite, Nutril and Carnos make good additions to stock for flavouring soups and gravies.

In this kind of cookery there is no waste, all the food is edible and anything that remains over from dishes can be put together and made into curries, stews, cottage pie, etc., etc.

Excellent Salads can be made by the addition of uncooked scraped and sliced carrots and beetroot; and also by chopping up very finely celery, Brussels sprouts, French beans, green peas, cabbage, parsley, onions, etc. The bright colours of these raw vegetables are most useful in decorating galantines and other cold dishes, and when arranged with regard to colour, make a most artistic garnishing and are most wholesome.

Pea nuts, pine kernels, and hazel nuts are much improved in flavour by being put in a baking pan in the oven until slightly browned.

Lemon juice is a good substitute for vinegar in all sauces.

For making a smooth soup it is a good plan to rub the vegetables after they are cooked through a very fine hair sieve.

In making cutlets a stick of macaroni should be inserted in the thin end of the cutlet to represent a bone, it may be fried or not with the cutlet.

UNFIRED AND VITAL FOODS.

The following practical information and suggestions will be found helpful by those who wish to test the advantages of living solely upon uncooked foods—as now recommended by so many progressive physicians, dietetic specialists, and teachers of hygiene. Although such a strictly simple and natural dietary may at first involve some gustatory self-denial, the benefits resulting from its use are declared by many who speak from personal experience to be well worthy of any inconvenience or sacrifice involved.

List of Foods and Fruits. etc., that can be eaten uncooked.

Cheeses—Camembert, Cheddar, Cheshire, Cream, Dutch, Gorgonzola, Gruyère, Gloucester, Half-cheese, Pommel, Port Salut, Stilton, St. Ivel, Wenslet, Wensleydale, Wiltshire, etc.

Fruits—(Dried) Apples, apricots, currants, dates, figs, muscatels, peaches, prunes or French plums, pears, raisins, sultanas, etc.

(Fresh) Apples, bananas, blackberries, currants, cantaloupes, cherries, damsons, gooseberries, greengages, green figs, lemons, melons, mulberries, nectarines, orange, pineapple, pears, peaches, plums, pomegranates, quince, raspberries, strawberries, tangerines, etc.

Nuts—(Fresh) Almonds, Barcelona, Brazil, cobs, coconuts, filberts, Spanish, walnuts, etc. (Shelled) Almonds, Barcelona, cashew, hazel, pea-nut, pine kernels, walnuts, etc.

Roots—Artichokes, carrots, parsnips, turnips and potatoes (which must be very finely grated).

Vegetables—Cabbage (red and white), cauliflower, corn salad, cucumber, celery, chicory, endive, lettuce, leeks, mustard and cress, onion, parsley, radishes, sprouts, spinach, salsify, seakale, tomatoes, watercress, etc.

RECIPES.

Nut-meat—2-ozs. shelled nuts, 1-oz. bread, 1 tablespoonful of milk. Put nuts and bread through a nut-mill. Mix together with milk. Roll out thin and cut into shapes with glass. This is sufficient for two. Look well over nuts before using, do not blanch almonds but rub them well with a cloth.

Unfired Pudding or Cakes—1-oz. each of dates, sultanas, currants, candied peel and French plums, and 2-ozs. nuts. Put all through a nut-mill and mix well together. Roll out and make into cakes. For a pudding, put mixture in a well greased basin, press down, leave for an hour or so and turn out. If too moist add breadcrumbs. Serve with cream.

Unfired Dried Fruit Salad—Ingredients as for pudding, but do not put through a mill; chop all the fruit and nuts and serve dry with cream.

Dried Fruits, such as French plums, peaches or apricots should be put in soak for 12 hours. Do not cook.

SALADS.

Brussels Sprouts—Use hearts only, which cut into small pieces.

Cabbage—Use hearts only, which cut into small pieces.

Cauliflower—Use flower part only, which cut into small pieces.

Chicory or Seakale—Cut into small pieces.

Lettuce—In the usual way.

Spinach and Mint—Use leaves only, which cut up very small.

Root Salad—Carrots or beetroot and turnips. Peel and put through a nut-mill and mix well together.
Most green salads are improved with the addition of radishes.
Salads can be mixed ad lib., but a greater variety of food is secured by using one or two vegetables only at a time.

Salad Dressing—(1) Half a cup of oil, 1 tablespoonful of lemon juice and the yolk of an egg. Mix egg with oil and add lemon afterwards. (2) Half a cup of oil and one well mashed tomato mixed well together.

Flavourings—For Nut-meat—Use grated lemon peel, mint, thyme or grated onion. For Dried Fruit Pudding or Cake—Use ground cinnamon, grated lemon peel, nutmeg, ground or preserved ginger.

QUANTITIES.

First meal at 11 o'clock—Per Person—approximately—

2-ozs. cheese.	3-ozs. salad or root salad.
2-ozs. dried Fruit.	2-ozs. brown bread, biscuits or unfired bread with butter.

Second meal at 7 o'clock—

2-ozs. nut-meat.	3-ozs. salad.
6-ozs. raw fruit.	2-ozs. brown bread, biscuits or unfired bread and butter.

It is well to drink only between meals, i.e., first thing in the morning after dressing; between first and second meal; and before going to bed. No alcohol or strong tea and coffee should be taken.

SOME SUGGESTIVE MENUS.

Spring—(March-April-May.)

FIRST MEAL.

SUNDAY—Tomato and Onion Salad. Cheese (St. Ivel). Unfired Pudding and Cream.

MONDAY—Carrot and Beetroot Salad. Cheese (Pommel). Dried Figs.

TUESDAY—Onions. Cheese (Cheddar). Dates.

WEDNESDAY—Seakale Salad. Cheese (Gruyère). Raisins.

THURSDAY—Salsify Salad. Cheese (Camembert). Sultanas.

FRIDAY—Celery Salad. Cheese (Wiltshire). French Plums.

SATURDAY—Batavia. Cheese (Cheshire). Dried Apricots.

SECOND MEAL.

SUNDAY—Cucumber Salad. Nut-meat (Jordan Almonds). Fresh Fruit Salad.

MONDAY—Endive Salad. Nut-meat (Hazel). Apples.

TUESDAY—Spring Cabbage Salad. Nut-meat (Pine Kernels). Oranges.

WEDNESDAY—Corn Salad and Radishes. Nut-meat (Cashew). Red Bananas.

THURSDAY—Watercress and Radishes. Nut-meat (Shelled Walnuts). Tangerines.

FRIDAY—Spinach and Mint Salad. Nut-meat (Barcelona). Bananas (Canary or Jamaica).

SATURDAY—Cauliflower Salad. Nut-meat (Peanuts). Fresh Cape Fruit.

Summer—(June-July-August.)

FIRST MEAL.

SUNDAY—Tomato and Parsley Salad. Cheese (Dutch). Peaches.

MONDAY—Carrot and Turnip Salad. Cheese (Cream). Apples.

TUESDAY—Spring Onion Salad. Cheese (Cheddar). Plums.

WEDNESDAY—Endive (summer) Salad. Cheese (Half-cheese). White Currants.

THURSDAY—Cabbage Lettuce Salad. Cheese (Stilton). Pears.

FRIDAY—Seakale Salad. Cheese (Gorgonzola). Banana.

SATURDAY—Corn Salad & Radishes. Cheese (Gloucester). Raspberries.

SECOND MEAL.

SUNDAY—Cucumber Salad. Nut-meat (Pine Kernels). Fresh Fruit Salad.

MONDAY—Lettuce Salad. Nut-meat (Cashew). Strawberries.

TUESDAY—Watercress and Radishes. Nut-meat (Almonds). Red Currants.

WEDNESDAY—Summer Cabbage Salad. Nut-meat (Shelled Walnuts). Greengages.

THURSDAY—Cauliflower and Mustard and Cress. Nut-meat (Hazels). Gooseberries.

FRIDAY—Mixed Salad. Nut-meat (Barcelona). Black Currants.

SATURDAY—Lettuce and Radishes. Nut-meat (Peanuts). Cherries.

Autumn—(September-October-November.)

FIRST MEAL.

SUNDAY—Tomato Salad. Cheese or Fresh Almonds. Pineapple.

MONDAY—Carrots and Celery. Cheese or Fresh Cob Nuts. Damsons.

TUESDAY—Corn Salad and Radishes. Cheese or Filberts. Apples (Golden Nobs).

WEDNESDAY—Brussels Sprouts Salad. Cheese or Barcelona Nuts. Melon.

THURSDAY—Onion Salad. Cheese or Brazil Nuts. Grapes (White).

FRIDAY—Endive Salad. Cheese or Fresh Walnuts. Bananas.

SATURDAY—Red Cabbage. Cheese or Hazel Nuts. Pears.

SECOND MEAL.

SUNDAY—Cucumber Salad. Nut-meat (Almonds). Fresh Fruit Salad.

MONDAY—Chicory Salad. Nut-meat (Hazel). Grapes (Black).

TUESDAY—Cabbage Lettuce Salad. Nut-meat (Pine Kernels). Pears.

WEDNESDAY—Celery. Nut-meat (Walnuts). Green Figs.

THURSDAY—Cauliflower Salad. Nut-meat (Cashew). Blackberries.

FRIDAY—Watercress and Radishes. Nut-meat (Barcelona). Quince.

SATURDAY—White Cabbage Salad. Nut-meat (Peanuts). Apples.

Winter—(December-January-February.)

FIRST MEAL.

SUNDAY—Tomato and Celery Salad. Cheese or Fresh Almonds. Dried Fruit Salad.

MONDAY—Carrots and Artichokes. Cheese or Cob Nuts. Dried Figs.

TUESDAY—Onions. Cheese or Fresh Walnuts. Dates.

WEDNESDAY—Batavia. Cheese or Brazil Nuts. Raisins.

THURSDAY—Cauliflower Salad. Cheese or Filberts. Sultanas and Currants.

FRIDAY—Red Cabbage Salad. Cheese or Barcelona Nuts. French Plums.

SATURDAY—Mixed Root Salad. Cheese or Spanish Nuts. Dried Peaches.

SECOND MEAL.

SUNDAY—Cucumber Salad. Nut-meat (Pine Kernels). Fresh Fruit Salad.

MONDAY—Celery Salad. Nut-meat (Hazel). Oranges.

TUESDAY—Winter Cabbage. Nut-meat (Almonds). Bananas.

WEDNESDAY—Corn Salad & Radishes. Nut-meat (Walnuts). Grapes.

THURSDAY—Cabbage Lettuce Salad. Nut-meat (Cashew). Red Bananas.

FRIDAY—Chicory Salad. Nut-meat (Peanuts). Tangerines.

SATURDAY—Endive Salad. Nut-meat (Barcelona). Apples.

The above Menus are compiled by the Misses Julie and Rose Moore.

USEFUL DOMESTIC INFORMATION.

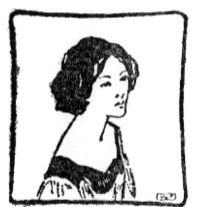

A clove of garlic will give a very delicate and tasty flavour to many soups and other dishes. For soups it is only necessary to rub the tureen with the cut clove before the soup is poured in. For savoury dishes and stews one small clove may be boiled (after being peeled) in the stewpan for five minutes.

To remove the skins from tomatoes place them in boiling water for about two minutes.

Turnips taste much better if a little cream is added to them after being mashed.

Any cold green vegetable can be used to make a soufflé. It should be rubbed through a sieve, and then 1 or 2 well-beaten eggs should be added. A few drops of Tarragon vinegar may be used to change the flavour. (See Recipe 97).

Cheese should be crumbly, as it is then more easily digestible. It is a good plan to test it in the following manner:—First buy a small piece and melt a portion with milk in a double saucepan; if it has a granulated appearance it is safe to buy some more of the same cheese; if, on the contrary, it is tough and stringy, it should be avoided, as it will be found lacking in nutriment and will be very liable to cause digestive troubles.

Butter should be made to look dainty and appetising by being prepared for the table with butter pats. Small pieces can be twisted round to form the shape of a hollow shell. It may also be rolled into marbles and be garnished with parsley.

Parsley can be made a brilliant green by placing it in a cloth (after chopping), dipping it in cold water, and wringing it tightly in the hands, squeezing it with the fingers. For garnishing savoury puddings or fried potatoes, etc., this is worth knowing.

Parsley which has been used for garnishing, or which is in danger of going to seed, can be preserved green for seasoning purposes by placing it in the oven on a sheet of paper, and drying it slowly in such a manner that it does not burn; it should then be rubbed through a sieve and put into a bottle.

All boiled puddings should be allowed room to swell, or they may prove heavy when served.

Instead of chopping onions, a coarse nutmeg grater should be kept for the purpose, and the onion should be grated like lemon rind. This saves much time and labour and answers better for flavouring soups, gravies, or savouries of any kind.

The addition of some bicarbonate of soda to the water in which onions are boiled will neutralize the strong flavour of the oil contained in them, and prevent it from becoming troublesome to those with whom it disagrees.

Freshly cut vegetables are more digestible and wholesome than those which have been lying about in crates or shop windows. They also cook more quickly. The water in which vegetables have been boiled should be saved for stock for soups and gravies (except in the case of potatoes).

To prevent hard-boiled eggs from becoming discoloured, they should be plunged into cold water as soon as they are removed from the saucepan.

Those of my readers who wish to use unfermented and saltless breads and cakes can obtain the same from the Wallace P. R. Bakery. The purity of goods supplied from this factory can be depended upon.

When it is difficult to obtain pineapples for making fruit salads, the same enhanced flavour can be secured by adding some of Dole's Hawaiian Pineapple Juice.

To prevent the odour of boiled cabbage pervading the house, place a piece of bread in the saucepan.

Flaked nuts, if sprinkled over puddings, custards, trifles or jellies, greatly improve the flavour and appearance.

In the preparation of soups, stews, &c., the preliminary frying of the vegetables improves the flavour and dispenses with any insipidity. The oil should be fried until it is brown.

HOW TO COOK VEGETABLES.

Artichokes should be boiled until tender only. If over-boiled they become dark coloured and flavourless.

Asparagus should be cut into equal lengths and tied into bundles. These should be stood on end in a deep stewpan, leaving the tops about an inch above the water. When the stalks are tender the tops will be cooked also. This plan prevents the tops falling off through being over-cooked.

Cabbage should only be boiled until tender; if over-cooked it is pulpy and flavourless. Boiling too fast causes the unpleasant odour to be given off which is sometimes noticeable in a house when this vegetable is being cooked. The lid of the saucepan should not be used.

Cauliflower must not be boiled until its crispness is lost. It must be only just tender enough to eat. It can be served 'au gratin' (120), or as in recipe No. 121.

Carrots should be steamed, not boiled. The skins should then be wiped off and they should be served with a white or brown gravy. They are also nice if scraped, sliced and stewed in haricot broth (recipe 239). The smaller the carrots the more delicate will the flavour be.

Kidney or Haricot Beans need to be carefully trimmed so that all stringy parts are cut away. They should be boiled until tender, and no longer, and served with thin white sauce. The smaller and greener they are the better.

Old pods should remain unpicked until nearly ripe, when the solid beans can be used for haricot soup or entrées. The 'Czar' bean is the best to grow; it is the giant white haricot, and the seeds are delicious when picked fresh and cooked at once. There is the same difference between fresh and dried haricots, as between green and dried peas. Dried Haricots must be soaked in cold water for twelve hours before being cooked. They can then be stewed until tender—the water being saved for soup or stock.

Vegetable Marrow should be steamed or boiled in its jacket. The flavour is lost if this is removed before cooking.

Mushrooms should be fried very slowly in a small quantity of butter. They should be stirred during the process, and the heat employed must be very moderate indeed or they will be made tough. They can also be stewed, and served in the gravy when thickened with arrowroot.

Potatoes should be cooked in their jackets. To boil them in the best way, the water in the saucepan should be thrown away when they have been boiled for 5 minutes and cold water should be substituted. This plan equalises the cooking of the interior and exterior of the potatoes. When cooked they should be drained, a clean cloth should be placed over the pan and they should stand on the hot plate to dry. They should be lifted out separately, and should be unbroken and floury. Sodden potatoes ought to be regarded as evidence of incompetency on the part of the cook.

Potatoes baked in their jackets are considered by many to be preferable, and, as it is almost impossible to spoil them if this plan is adopted, it should be employed when the cook is inexperienced.

Fried potatoes, cooked in the Devonshire fashion, are nice for breakfast. It is best to remove some from the stewpan when half cooked on the previous day. These should be cut up in a frying pan in which a fair amount of butter has been melted, and the knife should be used while they cook. In a few minutes the potatoes should be well packed together, so that the under-side will brown; an inverted plate should then be pressed on them and the pan should be turned upside down while the plate is held in position with one hand. A neat and savoury-looking dish will thus be made, but over-cooking must be avoided previous to the browning process, or they will look sloppy.

Potatoes can be mashed with a little milk and butter. They should then be packed into a pretty shape and garnished with chopped parsley (109).

Another way of cooking them is to use the frying basket and dip them in very hot Nutter. They should either be cut into thin fingers previously, or else be half boiled and broken into pieces. This latter plan is perhaps best of all, and they are then termed "potatoes sauté," and are sprinkled with chopped parsley before being served.

A very savoury dish can be made by boiling some potatoes until nearly tender, and then putting them in a pie dish with small pieces of butter sprinkled over them; they should then be baked until nicely browned.

To make potatoes *white* when cooked they should be steeped in cold water for two hours after peeling.

Peas should be placed in a covered jar with a little butter, and should be steamed until tender. No water is required in the jar. The pods, if clean and fresh, should be washed, slowly steamed, rubbed through a colander, and added to any soup or other suitable dish in preparation. Another method is to boil the peas with mint, salt, sugar and a pinch of bicarbonate of soda added to the water. Small young peas should always be chosen in preference to those which are old and large.

Spinach should be cooked according to the directions given in recipes 90 to 92, or 103.

Beetroot should be baked in the oven instead of being boiled. By this method the flavour is improved and the juices retained.

LABOUR-SAVING APPLIANCES.

Domestic work in the kitchen may be very much simplified and lightened if proper utensils are employed, and those who are able to do so should obtain the following appliances, in addition to those which are generally used:—

The 'Dana' Nut-Mill. This is used for making bread crumbs from crusts or stale bread; for flaking nuts and almonds, etc., so as to make them more easy of digestion, and nut-butter so as to make it mix more conveniently with dough when employed for making pastry and cheese—rendering it more readily digestible. This nut-mill may be obtained from G. Savage & Sons, 33, Aldersgate Street, London, E. C., and from Health Food Depôts (price 7/6). It serves the same purpose as a sausage machine as well.

A Frying-Basket is necessary for letting down rissoles, croquettes, cutlets, fritters, potato chips, etc., into the stewpan which is kept for frying purposes. The stewpan should be four or five inches deep, so as to avoid the possibility of the Nutter or vegetable fat bubbling over and catching fire upon the stove. Aluminium or nickel are the best metals.

A Raisin Stoner. It enables one to stone a large quantity of fruit in a very short time. Most ironmongers stock these machines.

A Potato Masher. Necessary for flaking potatoes and preparing haricot beans, peas, etc., for admixture in rissoles or croquettes. By this means the skins can be easily removed after they are cooked.

A Wire Sieve (about 1/8th-inch mesh). Useful for preparing spinach, and in many other ways which will suggest themselves to every cook.

A Duplex Boiler. For scalding milk by means of a steam jacket. It prevents burning, and boiling over. The **Gourmet Boiler** is a valuable cooking appliance of the same sort. Failing these a double saucepan is necessary.

A Chopping Basin—a wooden bowl with a circular chopper which fits it. This prevents the pieces from jumping off and lessens the time occupied. It is also less noisy and can be used while the operator is seated.

MEDICINAL AND DIETETIC QUALITIES.

As it is important that those who adopt a reformed diet should know something about the dietetic and medicinal value of the articles they consume, the following information may prove helpful:—

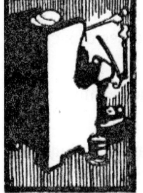

Apples purify the blood, feed the brain with phosphorus, and help to eliminate urates and earthy salts from the system. As they contain a small amount of starch, and a good proportion of grape sugar combined with certain valuable acids, they constitute a most desirable and hygienic food for all seasons. They should be ripe and sweet when eaten. People who cannot digest apples in the ordinary way should scrape them, and thus eat them in *pulp* rather than in *pieces*.

Bananas also contain phosphorus, and are consequently suitable for mental workers. They are easily digestible, and nutritious, being almost a food in themselves.

French Plums are judicious food for persons of nervous temperament and for those whose habits are sedentary; they prevent constipation, and are nutritious. They should be well stewed, and eaten with cream, Plasmon snow-cream, or Coconut cream (see recipe 224).

Strawberries contain phosphorus and iron, and are therefore especially desirable for mental workers and anæmic invalids.

Tomatoes are good for those who suffer from sluggish liver. The popular fallacy that they are liable to cause cancer, which was circulated by thoughtless persons some few years since, has been pronounced, by the highest medical authorities, to be unsupported by any evidence whatever, and to be most improbable and absurd. In the Island of Mauritius this fruit is eaten at almost every meal, and Bishop Royston stated that during his episcopate of eighteen years he only heard of one case of the disease.

Lettuce is soothing to the system and purifying to the blood. It should be well dressed with pure olive oil and wine vinegar (2 spoonfuls of oil to 1 of vinegar, well mixed together, with a pinch of sugar). A lettuce salad eaten with bread and cheese makes a nutritious and ample meal. The thin and tender-leaved variety (grown under glass if possible) should always be chosen.

Figs contain much fruit sugar which can be rapidly assimilated, and are very nourishing and easily digestible; when they can be obtained in their green state they are specially desirable. They may be considered one of the most valuable of all fruits, and are most helpful in many cases of sickness on account of their laxative medicinal properties.

Dates are very similar to figs, and are both sustaining and warming; they are easily digested if the skins are thin.

Gooseberries, **Raspberries**, **Currants** and **Grapes** are cooling and purifying food for hot weather; but, if unripe, they will often upset the liver. This type of fruit should not be eaten unless *ripe* and *sweet*.

Walnuts, Hazel and Brazil Nuts contain a considerable amount of oil, and are consequently useful for warming the body and feeding and strengthening the nerves. Vegetable fat in this form is emulsified and more easily assimilated than free animal fats, as in butter, etc. Nuts are also rich in proteid matter. Where people find that they cannot masticate nuts, owing to impairment of teeth, the difficulty may be removed by passing the nuts through a 'Dana' nut-mill. When thus flaked and spread between thin slices of bread and butter, with honey, they make delicious sandwiches for lunch. A pinch of curry powder (instead of the honey) makes them taste savoury.

Chestnuts contain a larger proportion of starch, but are digested without difficulty when boiled in their jackets until fairly soft. If eaten with a pinch of salt they make a nice dish.

Pineapples are valuable for cases of diphtheria and sore-throat, as the juice makes an excellent gargle. This fruit is considered to aid digestion in certain cases.

Cheese is very rich in protein—far more so than lean beef. If well chosen, and new, it is a most valuable article of diet, and feeds brain, nerves, and muscles; but as it is a concentrated food it should not be taken in excessive quantity. Half a pound of cheese is almost equal to a pound of average flesh meat. The best varieties are Wenslet, Gruyère (very rich in phosphorus), Port Salut, Milk (155), Wensleydale, Cheshire and Cheddar.

Protose, Nuttose, and similar malted nut-meats, are more than equivalent to lean beef—minus water, waste products, and disease germs. The International Health Association first invented these valuable substitutes for animal food, and has an able advisory medical staff, therefore they may be regarded as results of modern dietetic research. Protose contains 25% protein and 14% fat.

White Haricots are rich in protein (far more so than lean meat), and should be eaten in moderation. Brown haricots contain iron in addition to their large percentage of protein.

Lentils are almost identical in composition, but are more suitable for those who do not have much physical toil.

Peas are slightly less nitrogenous than lentils and haricots, but otherwise very similar; they are best when eaten in a green form, and when young and tender. When they are old the peas should always be passed through a potato masher, as the skins are very indigestible.

Macaroni contains starch and a certain amount of the gluten of wheat. Some of the best varieties are made with eggs as well as flour. Tomato sauce is the best accompaniment to it, with Parmesan or grated and melted cheese (see recipes 66 to 71).

Rice as usually sold consists chiefly of starch, but if unglazed and *once milled*, it is much more nourishing, as the cuticle of the cereal (which is rich in gluten and protein) is then left on it. The addition of cheese or eggs, makes it a more complete food (see recipes 72 to 80).

Potatoes consist principally of starch and water, with a certain amount of potash. Their dietetic value is not high.

Wholewheat Bread contains, in addition to its starch, much vegetable albumen, and a large supply of mineral salts, such as phosphates, etc. It is, therefore, when light and well cooked, of high dietetic value both for flesh-forming and nerve feeding. Physical workers should use it as a staple article of food, and mental workers will also find it most helpful. The coarser the brown flour, the more laxative is the influence of the bread. This is point worth noting.

Eggs are nutritive chiefly on account of the albumen which they contain in the white portion, but they are liable to cause digestive trouble, and they must not be taken too freely by those who are subject to biliousness and constipation. Such persons often find it advantageous to have them boiled quite hard.

Emprote (Eustace Miles proteid Food) contains the proteids of wheat and milk (35%), with digestible Carbohydrates (45.2%), fat (6.6%), and assimilable salts (7.9%). It makes a good addition to soups, beverages, and dishes lacking in protein.

Nuto-Cream Meat is a modern substitute for white meat and poultry, containing 19.7% protein, 48% fat, and 23% Carbohydrates. It is made from nuts and corn, and is useful for invalids and young children.

Milk contains nearly all the elements necessary for repairing bodily waste. It should be scalded for half-an-hour in a double saucepan—to destroy tubercular and other germs. If then allowed to stand for 12 hours, clotted cream can be skimmed off (as in Devonshire) and the milk can be used next day. It keeps much longer after being thus scalded. Dried milk is now procurable in such forms as 'Lacvitum' and 'Plasmon.'

Celery is a useful blood purifier, and is valuable in all cases of rheumatism, gout, &c. Celery salt is a valuable addition to soups and savoury dishes, and is preferable to common salt.

Spinach contains a considerable quantity of iron in a readily assimilable form, and is, therefore, good for anæmic persons.

Onions have a wonderfully improving effect upon the skin and complexion if eaten raw, and they act powerfully as diuretics.

HYGIENIC INFORMATION.

How to Keep Young. Old age is accompanied by the accumulation in the body of certain earthy salts which tend to produce ossification. The deposit of these in the walls of the arteries impedes the circulation, and produces senility and decrepitude. Flesh-food accelerates this process, but the juices of fruits, and distilled or soft water, dissolve out these deposits. The older one becomes the more freely should one partake of fruit and soft water.

The more juicy fruit we consume, the less drink of any kind we require, and the water contained in fruit is of Nature's purest and best production.

Frequent bathing and the occasional use of the vapour bath also help to eliminate these deposits, and those whose skins are never made to perspire by wholesome exercise in the open air must cause this healthful operation to take place by other means—or pay the penalty which Nature exacts.

Food and Climate. Vegetable oils and fats produce heat and build up the nerves. We require a much larger amount of food containing fat in cold weather and in cold climates than in warm weather and in warm climates. By producing fruits in profusion in the summer-time Nature provides for the satisfaction of our instinctive desire for such simple and cooling diet when the temperature is high. But in winter-time more cheese, butter, olive oil, or nuts, should be eaten every day.

Cancer and Flesh-eating. The latest declarations of some of the principal British medical authorities on 'Cancer' are to the effect that people become afflicted with this disease through the excessive consumption of animal flesh. The alimentary canal becomes obstructed with decomposing matter, toxic elements are generated and absorbed in the system, and cancerous cellular proliferation ensues. It is noteworthy that fruitarians are scarcely ever afflicted with this disease, and that a strict fruitarian dietary (uncooked) has often proved curative. See pages 133 and 166.

How to avoid Dyspepsia.

If the digestive process is unduly delayed by overloading the stomach, or by drinking much at meal-times so as to dilute the gastric juice, fermentation, flatulence and impaired health are likely to result. Raw sugar if taken very freely with starch foods is also apt to produce fermentation.

It is a mistake to mix acid fruits and vegetables by eating them together at the same meal. Fermentation is often thus caused, as vegetables take a long time to digest. A very safe rule to observe, and one which would save many from physical discomfort and suffering, is this—only eat fruits which are palatable in the natural uncooked state. Before Man invented the art of cooking, he must have followed this rule.

Those who suffer from dyspepsia will, in most instances, derive benefit by taking two meals a day instead of three—or at any rate by substituting a cup of coffee or of hot skimmed milk and a few brown biscuits for the third meal. Hard workers are the only persons who can really get hungry three times a day, and we ought not to take our meals without "hunger sauce." Fruit alone, for the third meal is better still.

The last meal of the day should not be taken after seven o'clock at night. Disturbed rest and the habit of dreaming are an almost certain indication of errors in diet having been committed, or of this rule having been infringed.

Probably the most valuable prescription ever given to a patient was that given by Dr. Abernethy to a wealthy dyspeptic, "Live on sixpence a day and earn it."

Constipation can nearly always be cured by adding stewed figs, French plums, salads, etc., to one's menu, by eating brown instead of white bread, and by taking less proteid food.

Tea is detrimental to many persons. The tannin contained in it toughens albuminous food, and is liable to injure the sensitive lining of the stomach. China tea is the least harmful.

Rest after Meals.

Those who work their brains or bodies actively, immediately after a solid meal, simply invite dyspepsia. The vital force required for digestion is diverted and malnutrition follows. The deluded business-man who "cannot spare the time" for a short rest or stroll after lunch, often damages his constitution and finds that he has been "penny wise and pound foolish."

If the brain or body has been severely taxed, an interval of rest should be secured before food is taken. It is not *what we eat* that nourishes us, but *what we are able to assimilate*. Recreation, occasional amusement, and an interest in life are necessary. Thousands of women die from monotony and continuous domestic care; multitudes of men succumb to mental strain and incessant business anxiety. Chronic dyspeptics should reflect on these facts.

Abstainers from animal-food who get into any difficulty about their diet should seek advice from those who have experience, or should consult a fruitarian physician. The local names and addresses of doctors who both practice and advise this simple and natural system of living, will be supplied upon application to the Hon. Secretary of The Order of the Golden Age. Such are increasing in number every month.

Physical Vitality.

The human body is a storage battery consisting of millions of cells in which the vital electricity that produces health, and makes life enjoyable, is accumulated.

Every manifestation of physical and mental power depends upon the force stored up in this battery. The more fully charged the cells the higher the voltage, and, consequently, the greater the physical vitality and power. This voltage is always fluctuating. Expenditure of force lessens it; recuperation, through rest, sleep, the in-breathing of oxygen, and the assimilation of vital uncooked food increases it.

Fruits, nuts, and root vegetables contain electrical potency—they will deflect the needle of a highly sensitive Kelvin galvanometer. But when cooked, their vital electricity is destroyed—they become *lifeless*, like flesh-food.

The accumulation of vital force is a possibility if natural and vital food is selected.

The Great Healer.

All the medicines in the world are as the small dust of the balance, potentially, when weighed against this Life-force—which "healeth all our diseases and redeemeth our life from destruction." Its therapeutic phenomena are truly wonderful.

When our bodies are invaded by malevolent microbes, the defensive corpuscles within us, if in fit condition, destroy them. But if not fed with those elements which are needful for their sustenance, they soon "run down"—just as we ourselves get "below par." We are then liable to become the prey of those ceaseless microscopic enemies that are ever ready to pounce upon the unfit.

If our corpuscles are weaker than the invading foes, no drugs can save us— we are doomed. Hence the importance of keeping ourselves and our nerve centres well charged and in vigorous condition.

How to Accumulate Vitality.
To accumulate vitality our food must contain all the chemical elements which we need. None must be permanently omitted. If, for instance, we entirely exclude organic phosphorus from the food of a man of great intellect, he will, in due time, be reduced to imbecility. This is obtained in such foods as cheese, milk, wholemeal bread, peas, apples, strawberries, and bananas.

We must live by *method*, and take some trouble. Nature's greatest gift is not to be obtained without thought or effort. We must eat, breathe, and live wisely; and the closer to Nature we get, the better it will be for us.

The habit of deep breathing, like that of living much in the open air, yields important results. The atmosphere consists of oxygen and nitrogen—the very elements of which our bodies are chiefly constructed. Life and vigour *can be inhaled*, but few persons have learnt the art.

Cheerfulness tends to promote the assimilation of food. Exercise—of an intelligent and healthful sort—is needful to make the life-current pulsate through our tissues. Without it our organs do not get properly nourished and rebuilt: stiffness and atrophy set in. Worry and care must be banished, and unwise or excessive expenditure of nerve force avoided; for these things deplete the human storage battery of its vitality.

Mankind is slowly gaining greater knowledge of vital, mental, and spiritual truth. Ultimately, "Life more abundant" will become the heritage of the many instead of the few.